PRAISE FOR

NEVER TOO LATE TO GO

VEGAN

"*Never Too Late to Go Vegan* shows the wonderful ways you can benefit from a new, healthier way of eating. This in-depth guide will inspire you to make the change and will hold your hand every step of the way, with all the helpful tips you need to make the transition smooth as can be."

—NEAL D. BARNARD, MD, author of *Power Foods for the Brain*
and director of Physicians Committee for Responsible Medicine

"What a wonderful book! If you want to be healthy, and to make choices that bring your compassion to life, this is your guide. Highly, highly recommended."

—JOHN ROBBINS, author of *Diet for a New America* and
The Food Revolution and cofounder of The Food Revolution Network

"*Never Too Late to Go Vegan* is a masterpiece created by an inspiring trio: Carol Adams, Patti Breitman, and Virginia Messina. If you are 50-plus and want to explore a vegan lifestyle, this book is an absolute must. It is incredibly informative and absolutely delightful from beginning to end."

—BRENDA DAVIS, RD, and VESANTO MELINA, MS, RD,
coauthors of *Becoming Vegan*, *Becoming Vegetarian*, and *Becoming Raw*

"What a terrific guide! Three wise women tell us everything we need to know to be happy, healthy vegans. This book is reason to celebrate and be well!"

—MICHAEL GREGER, MD, physician, author, speaker,
and director of Public Health and Animal Agriculture
at the Humane Society of the United States

THE EXPERIMENT

BECAUSE EVERY BOOK IS A TEST OF NEW IDEAS

"This is my new favorite book. Its nutritional know-how comes from science, not opinion. The recipes are tasty and healthy and unintimidating. Its ethical underpinnings arise from the real-life commitment of three wise women who were vegan before it was cool—and whose wit and savvy give me the feeling they've been cool all along."

—VICTORIA MORAN, author of Main Street Vegan and
director of the Main Street Vegan Academy

"Never Too Late to Go Vegan offers a warm, welcoming message to adults who have decided to adopt a vegan diet. Carol, Patti, and Ginny have combined their scientific knowledge and practical expertise to produce a book with a wealth of ideas for everything from eating well to social situations to caregiving. Simply put, this is an indispensable resource. Oh, and there are recipes too!"

—REED MANGELS, PhD, RD, coauthor of Simply Vegan

"An absolutely wonderful book, fascinating from beginning to end. Vegetarian for 20 years, vegan for 10, I still learned much from this terrific book! I intend to buy a dozen and give them away to inspire my friends who are over 50 to become vegan."

—JEFFREY MOUSSAIEFF MASSON, author of
Dogs Never Lie About Love and other best-selling books
on the emotional lives of animals

"If you think you are 'too old to change your diet,' that it is 'too late' or 'too hard to do,' or that you are 'too set in your ways,' you've got another 'think' coming! It is never too late and it's never been easier! This very comprehensive guide has gems of wisdom on every page—from demolishing prevalent myths about veganism, to how to make decadent, but healthy, desserts. Follow the plan in this book and you'll start seeing results tomorrow morning—and the rest of your longer, healthier, happier life!"

—RUTH HEIDRICH, PhD, author of
A Race for Life, Senior Fitness, and Lifelong Running

NEVER TOO LATE TO GO
VEGAN

NEVER TOO LATE TO GO
VEGAN

The Over-50 Guide to Adopting
and Thriving on a Plant-Based Diet

CAROL J. ADAMS
PATTI BREITMAN
VIRGINIA MESSINA, MPH, RD

THE EXPERIMENT
NEW YORK

The Experiment, LLC
220 East 23rd Street • Suite 301
New York, NY 10010-4674
www.theexperimentpublishing.com

The Experiment's books are available at special discounts when purchased in bulk for premiums and sales promotions as well as for fund-raising or educational use. For details, contact us at info@theexperimentpublishing.com.

The statements expressed in this book are not meant to be a substitute for professional medical advice. Readers should seek their own professional counsel for any health or medical condition before embarking on a new or different way of eating.

Library of Congress Cataloging-in-Publication Data

Adams, Carol J.
  Never too late to go vegan : the over-50 guide to adopting and thriving on a plant-based diet / Carol J. Adams, Patti Breitman, Virginia Messina, MPH, RD.
      pages cm
  Includes bibliographical references and index.
  ISBN 978-1-61519-098-0 (pbk. : alk. paper) -- ISBN 978-1-61519-185-7 (ebook : alk. paper)
1. Veganism--Health aspects. 2. Veganism--Social aspects. 3. Older people--Nutrition. 4. Vegan cooking. I. Breitman, Patti, 1954- II. Messina, Virginia. III. Title.
  RM236.A33 2014
  613.2'622--dc23
                              2013045262

Cover design by Christine Van Bree
Text Design by Pauline Neuwirth, Neuwirth & Associates, Inc.

Manufactured in the United States of America
Distributed by Workman Publishing Company, Inc.
Distributed simultaneously in Canada by Thomas Allen & Son Ltd.

First printing January 2014
10 9 8 7 6 5 4 3 2 1

To everyone over fifty making changes
for a better life and legacy

CONTENTS

PREFACE

With Age, Wisdom; with Wisdom, Vegan

GROWING OLDER ISN'T what it used to be. Active, inquisitive, open-minded adults of every age are following in the footsteps of younger generations who have turned to veganism with enthusiasm, commitment, and great results. Almost everyone knows of someone younger who is a vegan.

While college students get all the press for turning vegan in record numbers, those of us who are old enough to be their parents and grandparents need not envy them. We can join them and millions of others. It is our turn, now.

Change may be scary and challenging, but we've seen that before. We haven't gotten to where we are in life without change.

We wrote this book to reassure you, bust your notions of what aging looks like, show you how to prepare scrumptious food, and help you rediscover one of the most precious, life-affirming parts of yourself. We hope it will be a successful introduction to a lifestyle that brings you renewed energy, better health, a new sense of purpose, and a new experience of power to affect change. That is what it has done for us and for countless others who choose a vegan way of life.

Because we are all adults here, we are going to be honest with you. Sometimes that honesty will be refreshing, and sometimes it may be painful. But being vegan is a step toward being fully alive, and that includes being fully aware of life's beauty and sometimes its ugliness, too. With awareness, wisdom.

According to popular folklore, wisdom comes with age. What could be wiser than choosing compassion, vibrant health, and a vast, delicious cuisine to be the guiding principles in our life? Nothing!

That is why so many people are choosing to go vegan, or stay committed to their vegan ways when they are in the second half of their lives.

When we were in our twenties, thirties, and forties, our focus was most likely on raising a family or surviving at a job, building a career, or otherwise trying to make our mark on the world. But as we move away from the concerns of children and jobs, we wonder what are we moving toward? What habits have served us well, and what new routines might serve us better?

We (Carol, Patti, and Ginny) have lived a combined seventy-five years as vegans. We are eager to share with you the great news about being vegan after age fifty. Choosing a healthy, vegan diet helps reduce our risk of heart disease, stroke, diabetes, and perhaps cancer. Science continually confirms the myriad benefits of eating whole foods from the plant kingdom.

OUR VEGAN LIVES

How We Went Vegan

Patti: I never liked to cook, and I was a terrible cook before I became a vegan. In the early 1980s I worked for a New York publishing company, editing humor books and books about diseases. That provided a good balance because the books about diseases could be depressing, and the humor books perked me up. I still love a good joke, and jokes about food are my personal favorites. (Why did the tomato go out with the prune? Because she couldn't find a date! Sorry! My sense of humor is about third grade level.) When I edited Fit for Life by Harvey and Marilyn Diamond, I decided to try their program, which was about 98 percent vegetarian. I was wowed! Without cutting back on the quantity of what I ate, I dropped about 18 pounds in about six months. I had so much energy in 1985 that I trained for and ran the New York City Marathon, even though I'd never run more than six miles at a time before I started training.

Then in 1986 I moved to California, where people started asking me why I still ate eggs and dairy. "You have got to be kidding," I replied. "I made the biggest change in my life, and now you tell me that vegetarian isn't good enough? I have to give up dairy and eggs, too? No way!" But one person after another encouraged me to read *Diet for a New America* by John Robbins. He is the son of one of the founders of the Baskin and Robbins ice cream company. He is a wise man and a wonderful writer. That book opened my heart to the lives and deaths of dairy cows, laying hens, and every animal raised for food. Overnight I became a vegan.

When I discovered Jennifer Raymond's cookbook *The Peaceful Palate*, I first began preparing food that looked great, tasted delicious, and came out the right way every time. Now I find that I don't use recipes as often as I once did. I like to eat simply and improvise with whole, natural foods. When cooking for company I do use recipes, many of which are in this book.

Carol: I became a vegetarian in 1974 when I was twenty-three, after the death of my pony in a hunting accident. Two teenagers were target practicing in the woods behind our land, near where our two ponies were grazing. As their guns were going off near the wood's edge, Jimmy, our pony, collapsed. A neighbor who witnessed this ran to the house to alert me that Jimmy was lying crumpled on the ground. We ran together to the pasture and found Jimmy dead. That night, I bit into a hamburger and stopped mid-bite: What was the difference between eating a dead cow and a dead pony? Wasn't I a hypocrite if I only ate animals I never knew personally?

I realized that meat only exists because of the death of an animal. I decided to become a vegetarian. I knew that I loved to eat, and I didn't want to be tempted by foods I ethically wanted to give up, so I fasted on grape juice and water for one week. After fasting for seven days, I did not feel deprived by omitting meat and fishes because I truly appreciated all the foods that I could eat: vegetables, grains, beans, and fruits.

A year later I tried to be a vegan. But that was much harder. The soy milk in the mid-1970s was very beany in taste. It was hard to visit friends with their tempting vegetarian food. I abandoned that goal, only to have it reappear at the end of the 1980s when I was completing *The Sexual Politics of Meat*. I had coined the term *feminized protein* to represent such foods as milk from cows and eggs from chickens. It wasn't enough to analyze the problem of using these products that required the suffering of the animals. I knew I had to stop consuming them. Once again I had to figure out how to align my eating habits with my ethics. I began by giving up drinking cow's milk and experimenting with egg replacers. Cheese pizza was hard to give up at first, but as I looked at it, I brought to mind the suffering of cows who could not even walk to the slaughterhouse. I began to make our own pizzas and various vegan sauces (pesto, a white sauce, a Cheddar cheese–like sauce).

At the same time, I discovered wonderful vegan recipe books that provided alternative ways to prepare beloved family foods, such as lasagna, spaghetti Alfredo, moussaka, and spanakopita. Speaking on college campuses, I would ask the vegan students for their favorite recipes. I never looked back.

Ginny: I was one of those kids who was always bringing home stray puppies and injured birds—but it wasn't until adulthood that I made the connection between the food on my plate and the lives (and deaths) of animals.

I first dabbled in meatless cooking after reading *Diet for a Small Planet*, a 1970s book about the effects of meat production on the planet by Frances Moore Lappé. Dr. Lappé's perspective on food and the environment was absolutely groundbreaking and it opened my eyes to the fact that the effects of my food choices were far more impactful than just personal health.

But it was another several years before I made that leap of understanding about food and animals. I was a brand new RD at the time; that is, I had just passed the national exam to become a dietitian. I was also a newlywed. And while I wasn't exactly a novice when it came to cooking, I was enjoying the novelty of cooking for my husband and myself in our first home together. My cooking was taking on an experimental flavor as I explored new-to-me foods and dietary approaches.

One of my most valued guides was *Laurel's Kitchen*, a sort of countercultural vegetarian cookbook. I was standing in the tiny kitchen of my apartment in Kalamazoo, Michigan, on a fall evening when I opened the book and read: "This book is dedicated to a glossy black calf on his way to the slaughterhouse many years ago, whose eyes met those of someone who could understand their appeal and inspire us, and thousands of others like us, to give the gift of life."

Why those words hit me so hard is something I don't know. But they triggered a bit of an epiphany and I realized I was never going to eat animal flesh again. I became a vegetarian on the spot.

Six years later, when I was working for the government's National Cholesterol Education Program, I answered an ad in the classifieds of the *Washington Post* for a dietitian to work on vegetarian nutrition programs. Within weeks, I was working for the Physicians Committee for Responsible Medicine and was plunged into a brand-new world of plant-based nutrition. My co-workers were all vegans. I read *Animal Liberation* by Dr. Peter Singer and started becoming educated about animal rights. I learned about how dairy cows and egg-laying hens are treated on modern farms and began to steadily transition to a vegan diet.

It was a remarkable time in my life that set me on a professional path as a vegan dietitian that I had never imagined for myself. And more important, I'm forever grateful for the influences that led me to a lifestyle that brings me joy and a feeling of purpose every day.

Diets built around plant foods lower our risk for chronic disease. Even people with advanced disease can improve their health and reverse some symptoms with a diet based on whole grains, beans, fruits, vegetables, nuts and seeds.

And it's easier than ever to eat this way. We will guide you through a range of choices from simple ideas for meals to more elaborate choices for those who enjoy cooking. In fact, you've already eaten vegan meals. Do you ever have oatmeal with raisins and cinnamon for breakfast? Do you like peanut butter or almond butter sandwiches? Have you ever enjoyed pasta primavera with marinara or in a white wine sauce with garlic? And what about a hearty salad with arugula, fennel, chickpeas, and spinach? Or a mango-strawberry smoothie on a hot day? When you take inventory of some of your favorite foods, you'll see that vegan meals aren't quite as foreign as you may have thought.

We are going to show you how to adopt a vegan diet and thrive on it. There are so many ways to do this that you will find you can do it in any manner that feels right for you. You don't need to rethink everything. We will show you how to "veganize" your favorite foods and how to tweak family standards to make them vegan. We will show you how to minimize kitchen time and be able to have a dinner ready to serve in less than twenty minutes every day. If you don't like to cook, in chapter 8 we will explain how to order at restaurants. Beyond scrumptious recipes and time-saving food tips, *Never Too Late to Go Vegan* will support you in your veganism by focusing on physical changes, cultural stereotypes, nutritional needs, and social issues that are specific to people in their fifties, sixties, seventies, and beyond.

Until now, while there were scores of books for vegans of all stripes, none addressed the concerns and interests of mature vegans. We want to rectify that because one of the things we know is *with age, wisdom; with wisdom, vegan.*

PART ONE

IT REALLY *IS* NEVER TOO LATE TO GO VEGAN

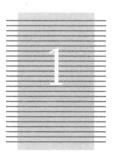

WHY NOW?
POSITIVE AGING THE VEGAN WAY

PEOPLE ARE LIVING longer and enjoying a variety of life experiences that their counterparts last century did not. On the other hand, aging as portrayed in our society is not pretty. Despite the movers and shakers who are fifty-plus, greeting cards and jokes about people over fifty, sixty, or seventy depict us as over the hill, past our prime, in our dotage, senile, foolish, useless, out to pasture, incapable, irrelevant, and worse.

The culture of youth is powerful. Advertisements often fixate on youth and circulate the attitude that looking young is the most important thing. Popular culture seems to imagine that as we age, we long for our youth again. It is presumed that we look backward, not forward. If this were ever the case, it certainly is not true now.

We are discovering how aging is about embracing change, and recognizing many of the freedoms that can come with getting older. We want you to know that veganism can help in the aging process, and that it really is never too late to go vegan.

• • •

FEELINGS THAT ACCOMPANY AGING: POWERFUL OR POWERLESS?

Aging may make us feel less powerful in relationship to our body and in our lives, and maybe less able to have an influence in the world.

THE 50-PLUS BODY

Have you ever heard a friend your age say to you, "Oh well, that just comes with aging." Do you buy into the notion that once we are past fifty we should expect a gain in weight and a decline in our health?

Aging may make us feel that we have less control over what is happening to our body. Our body shape surprises us. The aches and pains and illnesses we mention to friends—sometimes called the organ recital—seem out of our control. We seldom appreciate our health until we or someone we know is not well.

We propose that what are commonly thought of as diseases of aging (cancer, heart disease, diabetes) are no such thing. They are often the result of lifestyle choices over many decades that increase our odds of getting sick. So many of us fear getting sick, but until now did not have a workable plan for staying well. A well-planned vegan diet can reduce the odds of getting many of these diseases even as we age.

Some changes truly are related to aging: Our vision changes, our sense of balance changes, our taste buds change. But what seems to be prompted by aging may sometimes be the result of the food choices we have made over the years. The diet that most of us grew up on, sometimes referred to as SAD, for "Standard American Diet," is one that promotes a long list of health problems, such as clogged arteries, diabetes, digestive disorders, gout, constipation, cancer, and obesity.

Some of these diseases are far less common in cultures where meals are built around plant foods. It's not surprising. Plants provide fiber, for one thing, and they are also sources of antioxidants. Fruits and vegetables are especially rich in antioxidants and they also provide thousands of other types of phytochemicals that can help our body thrive and stay well. Phytochemicals are not essential nutrients; that is, they are not required for life. But they appear to have extensive benefits that protect and promote good health. In addition, whole grains, such as rice, wheat, quinoa, oats, and barley are full of fiber that helps lower blood cholesterol and keeps the intestines healthy. Nuts and seeds offer up healthy fats, including some that are essential nutrients and others that reduce risk for heart disease. Finally, legumes, such as lentils, chickpeas, kidney beans, black beans, soybeans, and white beans, provide the perfect combination of fiber, protein, and slowly digested starches to help lower blood cholesterol and promote feelings of satiety and satisfaction after a meal.

The good news is that when we replace old health-depleting food habits with new life-supporting food habits, we may find that our energy, cholesterol, and blood pressure will return to their natural, healthy levels. Some people see changes in weight as well.

EMPOWERMENT

> "My change to a vegan diet is permanent. It is part of a lifestyle change. I have also gone back to a natural hairstyle (I'm African American) and have added more Afro-centric pieces of clothing to my wardrobe. It all feels right for me at this point in my life." —DIANNE (61)

As we age, our sense of empowerment may change. We may feel that the kind of influence we had in the past has constricted. Empowerment, however, is double sided: it includes both influence on the outer world, and an inner feeling of being enabled to act. When something is not right in your world, whether it is your own health or the condition of the planet, you can simmer with anger (which is not good for you!) or you can find a way to take action to change things. Before you can act, you have to believe in your right to assert yourself, to believe that you *can* influence and change things. Too many people relegate that role to young people. Veganism is one way of empowering ourselves to respond to urgent issues in the world and to our own concerns.

"When I turned fifty I had an idea of the kind of man I wanted to be in my fifties and I am well on my way to becoming that man. But the most fulfilling thing of all is the knowledge that I am not contributing to the suffering of nonhumans and that I am leaving behind much less of an environmental footprint by my actions. I couldn't be happier." —BILL (51)

Even though we have lived more than half a century, when it comes to eating, most of us are still running on the programming from our childhood. We believe that we are making our own choices when we eat fish or chicken, eggs, or milk, but, in fact, we have been deeply conditioned to think of these as nourishing foods. When we choose them today, we may be acting from our lifelong habits and conditioning more than from our own wise decisions. Becoming empowered means facing squarely facts about these habits and learning about their impact.

Veganism isn't so scary. You probably could eat five vegan snacks right now:

1. Select a piece of fruit.
2. Put some peanut butter on bread and top it with a sliced banana.
3. Roll up a leftover salad in a tortilla.
4. Pop some popcorn.
5. Open a can of chickpeas, drain them, and heat them in a toaster oven with a seasoning (salt, pepper, curry) of your choice.

See, you have just created five vegan snacks!

VITALITY

Vitality is the life spark, the flame within; vitality is life itself. It's not synonymous with fertility, or whether or not you had children. Vitality is the energy that makes you glad to be alive. It is a gleam in your eye when you see something delightful, as well as the ability to grieve fully and feel all of your emotions at appropriate times.

With vitality, we focus on what we are doing, not which doctors we are seeing.

> "[Going vegan is] the best thing I've ever done for myself. I'm extremely pleased with my choices. . . . My only regret was not learning and growing in this compassionate direction decades sooner." —BEA (59)

Vitality takes the focus off the disintegration of health, off what you are losing, and keeps the focus on what you have, what you appreciate, and what you are building. You may discover that veganism is the commitment that connects you again to the healthy, happy individual you have always sensed you are. You will also feel the energy and vitality that come from the integration of intention and action.

Imagine if our relationship to aging were different. What if we didn't buy into the myths of aging, but instead lived the second half of our life with purpose, vitality, meaning, learning new things, sharing what we know?

> "I have no doubt whatsoever that this is the right path for me, and acting on what I know is right is one of the things I am most proud of. Sometimes the most difficult decisions are the most worthwhile. I tried to teach my children to do what they know is right, even if it is difficult and although they are grown women now, it's still up to me to live by example." —CAROL (61)

Throughout this book you will read about people who switched to a vegan diet after they were fifty. Most of them believed they were unlikely candidates for making such a change, but once they did it, they were thrilled. Going vegan is an opportunity to bring a new perspective to your role in the world. It is a way to take the best of who you are and who you have become, and consciously apply it to your life in a way that benefits yourself, the planet, and animals. In doing this, you will likely reawaken the sense of being an agent of change that you have known in the past. Disciplines as diverse as science and spiritual practice are on your side. Nutrition science continues to confirm the health-promoting benefits of diets based on vegetables, fruit, whole grains, nuts, seeds, and legumes. All the major religions have kindness at their heart.

Dorothy Morgan and Donald Watson Introduce the Term *Vegan*

In 1944, the word *vegan* (pronounced VEEgan) was coined. A group was forming and needed a name. Donald Watson and Dorothy Morgan, members of the group, were at a dance, discussing the need for a word that denoted the kind of vegetarian who used no animal products. What if the first three and last two letters of the word *vegetarian* were taken to describe people who at the time were called nondairy vegetarians? Morgan proposed the name; Watson liked it, as did the other members. Morgan and Watson married, and along with twenty-three other people, they founded the Vegan Society in England. Donald Watson said, "The Society soon widened its aim to include all animal exploitation, in brief, to work for a new relationship with the rest of sentient creation in a symbiotic relationship if possible, to live and help live rather than to just live and let live."

While both Morgan and Watson were very involved with the Vegan Society, the latter's role as secretary, treasurer, and auditor brought to him the role of explaining the word and popularizing the Vegan Society. Born in 1910 to a meat-eating family, he became a vegetarian at age fourteen. In an interview with *Vegetarians in Paradise* in 2004, he said that one of the reasons he became a vegetarian was, "As a child seeing animals pushed through doors alongside butchers' shops to be killed, I once saw a cow and a calf enter together. I wondered later which one the butcher killed first." Eighteen years later, when he learned about "the biological mechanics of milk production," he became a vegan.

Donald Watson wrote, "Veganism is a philosophy and way of life which seeks to exclude, as far as possible and practical, all forms of exploitation of and cruelty to animals for food, clothing, or any other purpose."

A woodworker and teacher his entire life, Watson was a conscientious objector in World War II and lived to be ninety-five years old. In an interview in *VegNews* magazine shortly before he died, Watson expressed his pleasure that the vegan movement lives on. We do not know what year Dorothy Watson died. World Vegan Day is celebrated every year on November 1 to commemorate the founding of the Vegan Society. (Look for a celebration in a city near you next October or November.)

5 REASONS TO GO VEGAN TODAY

1. A year from now, you'll be glad you did. It doesn't matter how old you are today; you will be one year older next year at this time. Becoming vegan today will give you fifty-two weeks to feel great.

2. You have the best book in your hand to make the transition. This is the guide written for you.

3. Your nieces, nephews, grandchildren, and your neighbors' children will admire you. It's a hot trend for young people, and our age group has been missing out on all the great rewards of being vegan. These young folks can introduce you to vegan recipes and give you cooking tips.

4. You will amaze your doctor. Many vegans see a welcome change in their cholesterol, blood pressure, and bowel habits within a few weeks of making the change to a vegan diet.

5. In the time it took you to read this list, nineteen thousand land animals were killed for food in the United States alone.

Going vegan has never been as easy or as delicious as it is today. Today, there are all kinds of prepared vegan foods that make vegan eating simple. Many restaurants offer good food for vegans. And more vegan restaurants are opening every year, especially in major cities.

POSITIVE AGING

Miso is aged. Wine is aged. Balsamic vinegar is more expensive the longer it is aged. What is fermentation of cabbage into sauerkraut but aging helped along with salt and darkness? Aging is an important process not just for some foods, but for each of us individually.

A beloved book, *When I Am an Old Woman I Shall Wear Purple*, articulates the freedom we discover as we age to decide for ourselves what we want. We are less intimidated by cultural or family expectations. We've been there, done that. Most of us, as we reach our fifties remember those times when we compromised our own values because of pressure at work or home. We might have stayed silent when we should have spoken up, or stayed in an unfulfilling job or relationship. But aging helps to bring clarity; the clock reminds us to seize the moment and to act on what we want and what we believe.

As our birthdays move us further from that half-century mark, we may find a change in focus from getting *what we want* to appreciating *what we have*. People may begin to focus on well-being and gratitude rather than monetary wealth and what it can buy.

We can enjoy the rewards of whatever we have accomplished with our life so far. And, whatever losses we may have suffered, we know there is a better future waiting for us when our focus shifts from "What is missing?" to "What choices can I make today to help bring about healing and well-being tomorrow and in the future?"

The only thing we cannot do is have a different past. The future is very much dependent on the choices we make right now, starting with our very next meal.

In her classic book, *Composing a Life*, Mary Catherine Bateson proposed that the model that envisioned someone being educated, holding one job, and then retiring from that one and only job no longer held true. Today people might go through several jobs in their lifetime, might refashion themselves several times over. But not just young people. We are given a chance in the second half of life to refashion ourselves again, and because of our experiences in the first half of life, we have learned that our choices really do matter. If our modus operandi used to be, "I've always done it this way," now is the time to embrace the new.

Bronnie Ware, a hospice nurse, wrote a blog about what dying people regret. She listed the top five regrets she heard from those she talked with as she provided palliative care. Her blog was eventually read by 3 million people. Two out of the five top regrets of the dying are relevant to anyone who has thought about or is thinking about becoming a vegan.

The first regret was, "I wish I'd had the courage to live a life true to myself, not the life others expected of me." So many people have said to us, "I would be a vegan, except my spouse would never agree." Or, "If I were younger, then I'd consider it." But in fact, being true to yourself can start today. We are also true to ourselves when we choose our food consciously, not out of habit and conditioning. Being true to ourselves means we are willing to change old habits when they are no longer good for us and replace them with new habits that are much better. In the next chapter, we'll give you suggestions for how to become vegan.

Another regret was, "I wish I'd had the courage to express my feelings." If you are feeling fear about changing, or sadness when you learn about what is happening to animals and the planet, or envy at those who have embraced new ways of eating, there is something you can do about it. Veganism is one way people express their feelings about and dreams for the world.

If you have heard of someone becoming a vegan, and you wish you were young enough to do it, you are! You will never be younger than you are today.

5 THINGS TO ENJOY!

1. The colors in your shopping basket and on your plate. You will be delighted by how attractive vegetables and fruits are. People will comment on how pretty your groceries look.

2. Discovering that many of your favorite foods can be veganized. As we advise on pages 215–217, many recipes can be veganized. If you don't find your go-to dish in this book, search on the Internet for "vegan ___" and you will find many recipes for whatever you are looking for.

3. Tossing out the laxatives. A vegan diet is naturally high in fiber, so most vegans can say good-bye to prune juice and milk of magnesia.

4. Discovering new foods. Many people report that their diet became more interesting once they went vegan. They gravitated toward menus inspired by Indian, Japanese, Indonesian, Mexican, and Mediterranean cultures. They also found themselves exploring foods like tofu, kale, and tempeh, which they had never thought about eating before. Vegan food can definitely broaden your culinary horizons!

5. Meeting other vegans and making new friends. Have you noticed when you get a new gadget, you are very aware of others with the same model? You might talk to strangers about theirs and share delight or ask questions. Once you are eating as a vegan, you will find fast kinship with other vegans you meet. Discovering another vegan is like finding a family member. We are so excited to share our experience with others who are blazing the same path to kindness. Go to meetup.com to find or to start a local vegan group that meets to eat or socialize.

VEGAN FOR A CHANGE

We three authors believe that adults over age fifty can appreciate the beauty, power, and effectiveness of a vegan diet in amazing and unanticipated ways. We find that adopting a vegan diet—or maintaining it—can be an affirmation of wisdom in aging and that aging can be a full celebration of life through veganism.

This time of life is the ideal time for kindness to blossom. So many of us thirst for kindness, but until now we haven't found a way to quench that thirst regularly. Veganism is one way to express kindness.

And if kindness is too "touchy-feely" for your taste, consider veganism as a form of justice. The way we treat animals raised for food is an appalling injustice. As decent human beings we can do right by other living beings by not breeding, confining, mutilating, and killing them with no consideration for their desire to live. Veganism is a way to promote justice.

Imagine if reaching retirement age was just as exciting as entering high school or getting accepted to college. Imagine that this milestone is, like those, an opportunity to widen our perspective on the world, encounter new, interesting people and ideas, develop new skills, and share what we learn to help others. Veganism offers all of this, and it is yours for the taking whether you are still working or long into retirement. And in veganism, we believe there is something that ties together many of the aspects of positive aging.

We love how choosing vegan meals makes us feel. We love that our choices do not hurt animals. We love that the food we eat reduces the methane production that is a major contributor to global climate change. If aging makes people feel they have less influence and power in the world, veganism offers a strong rebuttal to that feeling.

TIME IS ON YOUR (VEGAN) SIDE

People so often say that they don't have time to become a vegan. If they just had more time, or if we would do the cooking for them, then they would "eat this way all the time."

But you'll see that the amount of time you spend cooking is really up to you. You might find that there is something inspiring about the vegan kitchen, that preparing meals feels as if you are doing something especially positive and beautiful with your time. A little extra effort spent in preparing vegan meals doesn't seem time consuming; it feels valuable, and nourishing to body and soul.

But if that's not you, if you're someone who wants to spend as little time in the kitchen as possible, don't worry. There are options for all different types of cooks (and noncooks). Take a look at the Laziest Vegans in the World (laziestvegans.com) for some ideas on great vegan convenience foods. You won't want to make these foods the center of your diet, but combined with some of the tips for fast food preparation that we offer in this book (see pages 267–270), they can make your vegan diet just as easy as you want it to be.

Additionally, most vegans learn how to prepare delicious food in a hurry. A peek into the refrigerators of many vegans might look like a deli counter with lots of great, prepared foods, just ready to arrange on a plate, heat, and eat. In just two hours a week you can prepare everything you need for seven nights of dinners and seven days of lunches. With a slow cooker, you can prepare even more easy meals throughout the week. This cuts down on cleanup time as well as prep time throughout the rest of the week. We crank up the radio, MP3 player, or Pandora on a Sunday afternoon and spend a few hours in the kitchen, where we pull together two or three soups and sauces, cut up veggies for the week ahead, and make big pots of brown rice and quinoa. During the week we vary those dishes by adding different condiments and seasonings.

Leonard Bernstein said that what a composer needs is a great idea and not quite enough time. Aging reminds us that things we might have postponed should no longer be postponed. Ideas about taking better care of ourselves, ideas about eating well that we have flirted with from time to time are ready now for a more committed relationship.

You are not the first vegan, but are part of a movement that has been growing for decades. In fact, you're not the first person to go vegan after the age of fifty, either. When Ginny posted a request on her blog for stories from people who had gone vegan after fifty, the response was a little surprising and very heartening. Within one day, she heard from more than one hundred people who had adopted a vegan diet in their fifties, sixties, seventies, or even eighties.

Our vegan community is a treasure trove of resources. There are hundreds of tips and hints, recipes, and ideas already in use, just waiting for you to adopt and adapt. You don't have to invent meals and menus from nothing. And you don't have to do it our way or any one way. There is a world of welcoming people who are eager to share their success with you. Time is on your (vegan) side.

VEGANS OVER 50 TELL THEIR STORIES

Like Daughter, Like Mother | Colleen Welsh and Sam Kelly

Colleen's story: "To me, being vegan is life changing; I feel so much more positive about life."

When Colleen, a schoolteacher, was forty-eight, a young vegan, Mary, joined her teaching team. While getting to know her, Colleen asked Mary why she had chosen to be a vegan. Mary started to explain the ethical issues associated with the production of meat, dairy, and eggs. Colleen had known some very militant vegetarians, and found their confrontational style a turnoff. Mary, however, was low key, suggesting websites and information for Colleen to consider.

Colleen always tells her students, "If you are unaware of something, that's okay. You're not held responsible for something you are unaware of. But when someone awakens you to information, it's your obligation to figure it out and make your own decisions based on what you find out." As an educator, Colleen felt her role wasn't just to give this advice, but to follow it herself. "I realized I needed to educate myself; ignoring information doesn't make it go away."

She began by researching factory farming. "When I finally sat and looked at what was happening to animals, I said, 'That is not okay.' It was a real awakening for me."

For Colleen, veganism was an ethical decision: "Once I understood what it meant to be a meat eater and where eggs came from and what happened to cows for there to be milk, I informed my husband, 'I am no longer eating meat, I will no longer buy meat, or dairy or eggs.'"

Her becoming a vegan in October threatened her family's ideas about what they would be eating at Thanksgiving and Christmas. She wasn't asking her family or friends to change; still, there was anger at her having changed.

It took her a year of talking with her family about the holiday traditions they followed: What does each feast represent? How can we honor what Thanksgiving represents without turkey? How can we really appreciate being together and celebrating? Instead of dyeing Easter eggs, she began a new tradition of decorating papier mâché eggs.

Now, Colleen serves her family "new favorites that are delicious, healthy, and festive." She has enjoyed opening her family's palate with international foods. One thing in her favor is that her grandmother, who was Italian, was the one who taught her to cook. Colleen has veganized those of her grandmother's recipes that weren't already vegan (see pages 299–301).

Meanwhile, Colleen discovered how to respond to invitations to dinner parties. When friends would say, "I don't know what to make for a vegan," she would offer to bring a main dish and would assure the host that she could eat the side dishes if they did not contain butter or cheese.

At first, restaurants were a challenge. "When I became a vegan, I didn't know how to help restaurants know how to serve me." She didn't want to be seen as a complainer or difficult.

But now Colleen has recognized how to be her own advocate: If she goes to a restaurant where the food is prepared onsite, she will explain that she doesn't eat meat, dairy, or eggs—and has discovered that people are happy to accommodate her. She proposes new meals derived from the menu: "Could I have all the vegetables from the omelet on top of the hash browns instead?" She recognizes now that if you just know how to ask, veganism is not a big impediment to your social life.

There was one more area of her life that she had to negotiate: convincing her doctor that going vegan was a good idea. Colleen's doctor "was really nervous when I told her I was becoming a vegan. She asked, 'Where are you going to get your protein from?' I really had to educate her as well as myself." Now, "Every year my doctor is amazed at my blood numbers, my cholesterol numbers. She says, 'Wow, you are just a walking billboard for living a vegan lifestyle.'"

Colleen continues, "I haven't a peer who doesn't constantly diet. Growing up in the 1960s and the '70s, I remember this whole fascination with dieting, with being thin. I never worry about what I eat. I don't measure anything. I don't worry about calories; I don't have to worry about it. I have a healthy relationship with food for the first time in my life. Now I just enjoy it. I would never jeopardize my health again."

Even her school has embraced veganism. It is an independent/private pre-K to ninth grade school that requires students to eat the school lunch. Teachers are provided with lunch as one of their benefits. When Mary and Colleen approached the chef about more choices for them, he was initially very resistant. They spent time talking with him and met with the school administrators to educate them and to stress this was also a diversity issue. The school strives to be an inclusive environment but had not considered how this extended to dietary choices. Mary and Colleen spent a school year devoted to relationship building and education. Now, the chef actively studies the nutritional needs of vegans and provides a vegetarian, vegan, and gluten-free option at every lunch. The school also includes vegan food at all school-sponsored events.

■

Sam's story: "It's a wonderful new adventure. That's the way I want to think about life now."

Colleen's mother, Sam, was widowed in 2004 when Sam was 64 years old.

Cooking was never Sam's forte. After her husband died, Sam realized she was eating badly: her dinners were wine and cheese and crackers or prepared foods, such as TV dinners. If she didn't feel like cooking, she'd make a bag of popcorn. But then she told herself, "You just can't keep doing this."

Sam had been learning about veganism through Colleen, who, by this time, had been vegan for three years. Inspired to change, Sam began by getting rid of "all the damn crap I had in the pantry." When she first read the ingredient labels of canned soups, she was shocked. Unlike Colleen, Sam had not really ever cooked from recipes, but Colleen sent her *The Complete Idiot's Guide to Vegan Cooking* and *Vegan Vittles*, and Sam began to try the recipes.

At the beginning of each month, Sam shops for nonprocessed foods and spends two days "anchored to the stove." She cooks big batches of soups and makes stir-fries and then freezes them. When she doesn't feel like cooking, Sam enjoys the convenience of reaching into her freezer for one of the healthy dishes she prepared at the beginning of the month.

She also has discovered that while she still doesn't like cooking, she enjoys salads. "You can make a cold dinner out of a salad, with tons of beans, and fruit and nuts. You discover different kinds of lettuce."

She is also thrilled with all the new tastes and flavors of a vegan diet. "I am not worried about the protein, because I have learned how many things without meat have protein. " She has seen her cholesterol, "which was getting toward 200," plummet, and generally doesn't take any medications.

About eighteen of her high school classmates (class of 1957), many of them widows, get together once a month. They respect her veganism. "They can be pretty supportive; at this age, we live and let live." One friend, who has type 2 diabetes, has also adopted veganism.

Her vegan lifestyle does not prevent her from traveling. Recently she's been to Egypt, Africa, China, and Scotland. She supports her travels by painting and selling small watercolors.

Sam has been following an almost complete vegan diet for three and a half years. "I have a great life; I have wonderful kids, nine grandchildren, and two great-grandchildren. I am just having the time of my life, because I am looking at the short end of the tunnel. So you want to maximize your days, you want to be involved with people, give of yourself to your friends, and enjoy as they give back to you; that's what I do! You've got to have goals, have something new in your life. You have to stretch yourself a little."

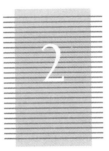

HOW TO GO VEGAN: YOUR NEXT MAJOR LIFE DECISION

WHILE WAITING IN a line, Annie Shannon, coauthor of the popular cookbook, *Betty Goes Vegan*, began talking with two women who were in their eighties. The first woman said, "I could never go vegan. I just feel like I would be turning my back on my mother's food." The other woman turned to her and said, "Someday you're going to have to decide to be your own woman."

While this sounds like a routine out of the television show *Golden Girls*, there is so much truth in the second woman's statement. But we want to go further: We want to suggest that your next major life decision is not *whether* to become a vegan, but *how*.

5 THINGS TO KNOW AS YOU BECOME VEGAN

1. **Becoming vegan is easier than you think.** There may be some challenges, but you're very likely to find that making the change to a vegan diet is easier than you thought it would be. Tastes change over time and you'll find yourself enjoying new foods as you explore them. And as those foods replace the familiar fare of the past, most vegans find that they sim-

ply stop thinking about the animal foods that were once part of their diets.

2. **Ingredients in vegan recipes are often optional and or substitutable.** Unlike a soufflé, vegan food is very forgiving. So don't be discouraged if you don't have exactly the right ingredient for a recipe. If you don't have a red onion, use scallions or a yellow onion or even dried onion flakes. If your recipe calls for French lentils and you have only regular lentils, that's okay. If you use oregano when marjoram is called for, your food will not suffer for it. Unless you are making a grilled cheese sandwich, you can usually omit the vegan cheese from vegan recipes, especially when it is intended as a topping, such as in burritos or salads. (If you *are* making a grilled cheese sandwich, see our chapter, "How to Veganize," page 215).

3. **Vegan food is delicious, but that doesn't mean you will love every recipe.** Patti has more than one family member who can't stand peanut butter. So she does not make her favorite comfort foods—peanut butter sandwiches and peanut sauce with pasta—for these people. No doubt, you'll find that there are some vegan dishes or ingredients that aren't your favorites. Just keep exploring and experimenting and you'll find plenty of vegan foods to love.

4. **Restaurants are usually accommodating and it's okay to ask for what you want.** We're not talking about McDonald's or Burger King here, but at most restaurants where a waiter comes to your table, the server is usually happy to relay your request to the kitchen. (Side note: Most waiters are not paid even a minimum-wage salary, but depend on tips. Please be sure to tip generously when you eat out, not only to help these hardworking people, but also to represent vegans as thoughtful, appreciative people.)

5. **Resources abound.** If you like to cook, you are going to have a blast in the kitchen. And, if you need reassurance, there are dozens of websites and hundreds of people who are happy

to share advice, recipes and techniques online. But if you don't like to cook, you can assemble foods and find takeouts—nothing has to be created from scratch (see "Easy Vegan Meals for the Noncook," page 267). And there are vegetarian versions of most meats, made from seitan or soy protein, tofu, or tempeh.

If you have only seen vegans eat in a nonvegan environment—a home where the host is not familiar with veganism—or a restaurant where you may have heard a vegan order only sides and salads with lots of instructions to the waiter, you may think vegans are deprived. Not so!

When we are in a vegan environment in our own home or someone else's, or when we visit a vegan-friendly restaurant, the choices are boundless. Vegan options abound in cuisines of the Mediterranean, the Middle East, India, Africa, Asia, Central and South America, and other areas where plant-based diets are common. Whether we frequent international restaurants or learn to use the herbs and spices that flavor their food (see pages 291–294), a whole world of new tastes and textures is waiting for us. And vegan restaurants are opening all over the country (and world), while many other restaurants are adding vegan items to their standard menus, as more and more people discover the benefits of this delicious lifestyle. (Visit happycow.net to find a vegan-friendly restaurant anywhere in the world.)

ADVICE AND INFORMATION FOR NEW VEGANS

In 2011, Patti and Carol conducted a survey focused on the question, "What do vegans eat?," to which they received more than two hundred responses. Many of the respondents said, "I wish I had known how easy it would be to be a vegan." One man, a sixty-seven-year-old, became a vegan after experiencing a health crisis. His daughter, a vegan, gave him vegan books. He simply called himself "the older guy who gets it!"

People noted how many resources and vegan products are available. One person reported, "The day I went vegan I thought, 'Crap: I have to be in Las Vegas for a work trip in three days. How on earth are you supposed to eat vegan there, where all the food is gobs of gross decadent stuff and everything is slathered in everything?' But, you know what? It wasn't even a challenge."

Even if you are the only person in your household who is going vegan, you don't have to do it by yourself. Find someone who is a successful happy vegan and ask him or her to help you transition. Having a vegan buddy is especially helpful if your family or co-workers are not supportive. Check for local groups at meetup.com, craigslist .org, or bulletin boards at the natural foods store or library. If you can't find a vegan group, consider starting one. You'll find support online as well. Vegan discussion forums, such as those at theppk.com or veganforher.com, can put you in touch with others in transition as well as with longtime vegans who can answer your questions.

Some people find that going "cold turkey," or, as we like to say, "cold tofu," works well. If you plan in advance what you will eat each day, going vegan all at once can be a fun adventure. Most people who do this say in retrospect that it was easier than they had imagined it would be.

Regardless of how you begin your journey to veganism, the following suggestions will help make the transition a smooth one.

10 WAYS TO GET STARTED TODAY

1. **Go vegan one day a week.** The popular Meatless Monday program that many cities, schools, restaurants, and companies are adopting encourages a meatless day once a week to reduce pollution and to improve health. To move toward veganism, simply choose one day, Monday or any other, and plan your meals and snacks for that day. This method cuts down on your intake of cholesterol and saturated fat, reduces your carbon footprint, and reduces the number of animals killed for food.

2. **Go vegan one or two meals a day.** If you eat a vegan breakfast or dinner every day, you will be starting or ending your day with a nourishing, health supporting meal. If you make vegan choices at both breakfast and dinner, you will be two-thirds of the way to being vegan.

3. **Eat vegan on weekends.** This is a great way to start if you work outside the house. Weekends are your own to experiment with recipes or try new restaurants. Think about vegan cooking as you would any cuisine new to you. You just have to learn a few new ingredients and techniques.

4. **Eat vegan on weekdays.** Weekday vegans set a good example for people at work. A thermos and cold box make it easy to bring vegan soups, salads, and sandwiches anywhere you go.

5. **Eat vegan at home.** Many people like to keep a vegan kitchen. Having staples on hand by creating a vegan pantry makes it easy to throw together a meal in no time. Throughout the book we suggest pantry options for vegans.

6. **Eat vegan when eating out.** Make it a habit to ask for vegan choices at restaurants. Even if nothing is obviously vegan, there are usually vegan sides that the chef can combine for a fabulous meal.

7. **Start by omitting a particular type of food.** Maybe you want to eliminate dairy or eggs first and then move on to finding substitutes for meat, fish, and chicken. (See the tips for giving up cheese, page 49.)

8. **Find recipes you already know and veganize them.** We offer an entire chapter on how to do this (see pages 215–234), but you could begin by replacing your nonvegan items with vegan ones: instead of sour cream, vegan sour cream; instead of cheese, nutritional yeast or vegan cheese (store-bought or homemade); instead of cow's milk, a plant-based milk; instead of hamburgers, veggie burgers. Replace meat with soy- or wheat-based analogues that have a texture and taste similar to that of animal-based meats. Tofu and seitan (wheat)

take on the flavors they are cooked with, so look for lots of different recipes for these ingredients (we provide some recipes on pages 230–234).

9. **Try one new vegan food or recipe every day.** Use this book or visit your library. There are dozens of vegan cookbooks in stores and thousands more vegan recipes are posted on the Internet. Pay attention in September, the Vegan Month of Food, for VeganMofo (see veganmofo.com), when bloggers gear up to write daily about the joys of vegan cuisine. If you are unfamiliar with a food, ask the staff at any grocery or natural foods store (Trader Joe's has a list of its vegan foods near its entrance). Also, if there is a farmers' market near you, visit and talk with the farmers. They usually know a great deal about the foods they are selling. Explore Indian and Chinese grocery stores and discover all the wonderful vegan foods there.

10. **Begin with vegan foods you already know and build from there.** Hummus, falafel, marinara sauce, minestrone, fruit and oatmeal, peanut butter and jelly sandwiches (of course!), and even some of the most popular mainstream products—for instance, Green Giant Cream-Style Sweet Corn, Oreos, Cap'n Crunch Cereal—are all vegan. You get the idea—you are probably already enjoying many vegan foods.

The best advice we can offer for going vegan is this: Don't focus on what you can't eat, but look at the many foods you *can*. In *The Ultimate Vegan Guide*, author Erik Marcus suggests, "Don't cut out non-veggie foods, crowd them out." If you are accustomed to eating chicken, fish, or red meat in the center of your plate, think instead about centering your meals around whole grains, potatoes, beans, or pasta (whole-grain pasta when possible). Then fill the rest of the plate with vegetables. Do you remember TV dinners, where vegetables occupied a tiny compartment on a tray? Never again will veggies be second string. Vegetables—steamed, baked, stir-fried, barbecued, or raw—can now be a main dish! A plate full of roasted veggies is lovely (see our Roasted Veggies recipe on page 280). Or try an assortment of steamed vegetables topped with Indonesian peanut sauce (page 304). Or give them a quick stir-fry in your own homemade curry sauce or one from a jar.

OUR VEGAN LIVES

Tips That Helped Us Become Vegans

Patti: When I first became vegan, I attended a monthly potluck dinner for vegetarians and vegans. Most of us wore jeans and T-shirts to these dinners, but one woman, Kay Bushnell, always dressed beautifully. She wore very stylish and tasteful outfits, and I was quite impressed that someone who looked so well put together and professional was a vegan. That made a huge impression on me. I was still working as a literary agent then and had to travel to New York frequently for business. Kay helped to make me feel perfectly comfortable being a vegan in business attire. Without knowing it, she gave me permission to dress however I needed to dress and to feel that tailored clothing was appropriate for a vegan. I still think of her with fondness and gratitude whenever I am dressed up for a special occasion.

Carol: The breakthrough for me as I became a vegan was the realization that tofu could be a cheese substitute. My friend Shirley Wilkes-Johnson sent me her tofu feta cheese recipe and that allowed me to make spanakopita and Greek salad. Discovering a tofu ricotta recipe ushered in luscious lasagnas and calzones. (We include recipes for tofu ricotta and tofu feta cheese on pages 223 and 222.) When my family went out for pizza, I began to leave cheese off the pizza I ordered (and ordered double veggies instead), and found that I didn't feel left out at all. Then I slowly examined my presumptions: does French toast need eggs? Experimentation showed the answer was no.

I knew what I was leaving behind, and so realized I needed to introduce into my life plenty of proof of what I was choosing instead. By going to vegan potlucks, reading recipe books, asking vegans what they ate, and experimenting in the kitchen, I balanced out what was left behind with the new and inviting things that I was learning to use.

I also involved my kids. When my children were young, we would often read through a new vegan recipe book along with the usual storybooks at night. We'd select recipes they wanted to try. The following days, they would help prepare the recipes they had picked. As they grew up, they helped me as I experimented in making vegan ravioli, stuffed seitan, macaroni and cheese, and a variety of desserts.

Because others—through their advice, encouragement, and recipes—had shown me what was possible, I soon discovered that I no longer had a desire to prepare anything but vegan meals.

Ginny: Although I love finding vegan versions of foods that I grew up with—and those are meals that give me a great deal of comfort—turning to international cuisines made me realize how easy it was to be vegan. Taking advantage of recipes for curries, hummus, Mediterranean beans and pasta, and Asian stir-fried dishes helped me see that vegan eating could be delicious, satisfying, and authentic.

In addition, letting go of meal-planning "rules" made it far easier to create satisfying vegan meals. I've never been a cereal eater, and I really like something warm and hearty for breakfast. So I rarely eat traditional breakfast food, but instead am likely to have a bowl of lentil soup or a veggie burger first thing in the morning.

Those two things—exploring new foods and plant-based cuisines, and letting myself redefine meals—made the vegan transition easier.

VEGAN MYTHS BUSTED!

There have been many misconceptions about veganism over the years. Now that you are embarking on your own vegan path, you may want to know the *real* story behind these myths.

MYTH #1: VEGETARIAN FOODS NEED TO BE "COMBINED" TO PROVIDE COMPLETE PROTEINS.

You don't need to combine proteins to ensure good nutrition. Many people, especially those over age fifty, remember when *Diet for a Small Planet* appeared in 1971. Frances Moore Lappé's book made excellent arguments against eating meat. But it also introduced the idea that vegetarian foods did not contain complete protein the way that meat did, and that vegetarians needed to combine vegetable proteins to ensure they were eating healthfully. She explained that eating grains and beans together was the best way to ensure that the amino acids in both would combine properly to make a complete protein. In her book, because she was a good and careful writer, Lappé went into great detail about combining protein. Unfortunately, many people took away from her writing that getting protein from nonanimal sources was complicated.

The food combining craze took off, and a generation of vegetarians strived to combine grains and beans at every meal. Two decades later, when science showed that this was not necessary—our body can combine amino acids from meals over the course of a day—the updated edition of *Diet for a Small Planet* refuted the earlier assertion that foods had to be combined to form a complete protein. Because so many more people read the original book than the revised book, the myth of food combining lives on. We talk about meeting protein needs on a vegan diet (it's easy!) in chapter 5.

Another version of food combining taught that fruit should be eaten only on an empty stomach, and that nothing except fruit should be eaten before noon. It was based on Natural Hygiene, a system developed in the 1800s that emphasized rest, clean air, emotional poise, and eating whole, natural foods.

In the twenty-first century, the arguments that plant foods must be combined in a certain way are obsolete. Sometimes vegans have fun combining different colors of vegetables or fruits to create a beautiful plate. But they are not compelled to do it for scientific or nutritional reasons.

MYTH #2: ATHLETES CANNOT BE VEGAN.

Another prevalent myth is that athletes need to eat meat. This is a misconception; there are dozens of well-known runners, body builders, triathletes, and others who prove it wrong. Numerous websites exist for vegan athletes; if you Google "vegan runner," "vegan cycling," and so on, you will find information and support.

> *"I've done three triathlons at ages sixty, sixty-one, and sixty-three. We're very healthy and seem to have plenty of energy for work and extra activities, and I love trying new vegan recipes! It's opened up a whole new world of cooking!"* —SUE (63)

Ruth Heidrich is a triathlete who wins gold medals in her age category (over seventy) on a regular basis. She has been a vegan for decades, ever since she was diagnosed with breast cancer in 1982. Carl Lewis, a nine-time gold-medal Olympian runner and jumper, says that he performed his best when he became a vegan.

You are probably not going to be competing in the Olympics or entering triathlons. But even if you are, know that a healthy vegan diet provides all the nutrients you need to be strong, to be healthy, and to win. Extra-active people may need more calories, and body builders may need more protein. But these needs can be met easily with plant proteins, such as beans and soy foods, as well as more frequent meals to take in more calories.

"As an athlete, I was a little concerned at first about the effect of a plant-based diet on my performance. I have not seen any bad effects and my health has never been better. I make sure that I eat a mostly whole-food diet, supplement where necessary, and get enough calories to sustain my athletic activities." —DEBBIE (55)

And while we are on the subject of athletes and veganism, let's just mention that the macho image of men grilling steaks in the backyard is so twentieth century! Smart vegans today know that grilling is a potent way of releasing the flavors of eggplant and corn, of enjoying veggie burgers and veggie shish kebab (skewers with, for example, pineapple, summer squash, eggplant, and tomato). In contrast, grilled meat is linked to risk for colon cancer.

MYTH #3: VEGANS HAVE TO WORRY ABOUT NUTRIENTS AT EVERY MEAL.

As vegans we do not have to think about nutrients at every meal any more than nonvegans have to do so. As you will see in chapter 6, we do need more of certain nutrients as we age and some nutrients deserve a little bit of extra attention. But if we are eating generous portions of beans, whole grains, nuts, seeds, fruits, and vegetables, and following the simple guidelines in chapter 5, we'll easily get the nutrients we need.

MYTH #4: IT IS TOO HARD TO BE VEGAN.

People think that it's too hard to be vegan, but it is not. It can be challenging, but it is more challenging to be stuck in old patterns that are not serving us well. It is hard to be sick, and hard to live in fear of change.

Veganism opens up possibilities, including very easy ways of eating. Your meals can be simple ones that take just minutes to prepare—refried beans from a can, rolled in a corn tortilla and topped with fresh tomatoes and avocado; pasta tossed with gently braised vegetables and toasted pine nuts; a fast and filling chili—Festive Quinoa (see page 297); fresh fruit (the original fast food); baked or steamed sweet potatoes with a dollop of vegan sour cream, and more. The recipes (as well as the recipe-less ideas) in this book will guide you toward simple and delicious meals like these. When you want to expand to more elaborate dishes, we've provided recipes for Neatloaf, Moussaka, a stuffed seitan roast, and many others. In addition, thousands more vegan recipes are posted on the Internet.

If you think being vegan entails too much chopping and shopping, see "Easy Vegan Meals for the Noncook" (page 267) for time-saving tips.

MYTH #5: IT IS EXPENSIVE TO BE VEGAN.

The most inexpensive meals on the planet are vegan. Ellen Jaffe Jones's *Eat Vegan on $4 a Day* provides many recipes for eating vegan on a budget.

If meat and dairy foods seem cheap, it's because federal subsidies keep down production costs. But even without that support, plant foods remain a cost-effective way to get protein and other nutrients. The Median Nutrient Rich Foods Index Score, developed by public health expert Dr. Adam Drewnowski, ranks foods based on their cost per hundred calories and their nutrient value. The foods that deliver the highest nutrient value for the lowest cost? Beans, nuts, and seeds. Buy them in bulk to save even more money.

If you have Indian or Chinese grocery stores in your neighborhood, they are often an inexpensive source of foods like tofu, leafy greens, and curry sauces. And don't overlook more traditional stores. Warehouse outlets like Costco are a goldmine of cheap vegan foods, such as tofu, pinto beans, walnuts, peanut or almond butter, quinoa, hummus, veggie burgers, and soy or almond milk. They're a great place to find less expensive fruits and vegetables, too.

It's true that fresh fruits and vegetables can be expensive, and that's often especially true in low-income neighborhoods. But that's not really a vegan issue. *Everyone* should be eating more of these foods. And there are ways to reduce your costs. A backyard garden can provide optimum nutrition at very low cost. Community gardens are being started in urban areas around the country to provide the opportunity for harvesting one's own plants. You can also grow a surprising amount of fresh vegetables in pots on your patio or deck. Farmers' markets provide local produce at modest costs. Or sign up to be a part of a CSA (Community Supported Agriculture) program. Join with neighbors to share a weekly delivery of fresh-from-the-farm veggies and fruit. Use the locator service at localharvest.com to find CSAs, farmers' markets, and food co-ops near you.

If you have a freezer, it's easy to preserve your garden's abundance for the winter. Otherwise, frozen vegetables from the grocery store are often less expensive than fresh, and they are just as nutritious.

5 THINGS TO ENJOY AS YOU BECOME VEGAN

1. **Sign up at nutritionfacts.org for a free, daily video from Dr. Michael Greger.** Dr. Greger is the director of Public Health and Animal Agriculture at the Humane Society of the United States. He combs the nutrition and medical literature for nutrition information and creates short films (1 to 4 minutes) to explain what science is discovering about our food choices. These are informative and motivating, and a wonderful, daily reminder about the healthiest choices we can make. Browse the web for other sites that deliver daily, weekly, or monthly recipes, news, and buzz about being a vegan.

2. **Create a jaw-dropping salad.** Forget about lettuce and tomatoes; that was the old days. There is nothing wrong with lettuce and tomatoes, but we've eaten those for decades, and it's time to try something new. Now you are going to put in more variety than you ever thought a salad could accommodate! Think fennel, carrots, celery, chickpeas, bell peppers, radicchio, red cabbage, corn, peas, sunflower seeds, chopped walnuts, or edamame—anything with color or crunch. You don't have to put these on greens, as they make

a beautiful salad on their own. Or you may choose to use a base of spinach, arugula, or lettuce. (See pages 254–257 for dressing recipes and salad ideas.) Dress only as much as you will eat at one sitting, as the dressing will age the salad more quickly.

3. **Find vegan versions of your favorite recipes.** Find a recipe you love and try a vegan version of it. Maybe we included one of your favorites in this book. If not, search the Internet and you will find lots of options. In chapter 9, Carol describes a time when two caregivers were preparing some food for her. They did a Google search for "vegan lasagna" and found a recipe that Carol swears was incredible. Despite being a vegan for decades, she discovered that the dish had ingredient combinations she had never heard of.

You might also grab a copy of Annie and Dan Shannon's *Betty Goes Vegan* cookbook. They veganized the 1950s *Betty Crocker Cookbook*! Talk about the best of all worlds: you can have the comforting familiar dishes of your childhood, but revamped for healthier, more compassionate meals.

It's never too late to discover new vegan foods even when you're a seasoned vegan.

4. **Notice how your diet ties in with the news.** When you hear about droughts, antibiotic resistance, climate change, or the health-care crisis, know that you are now part of the solution. Rather than despair over all that is wrong, you can celebrate that you are a living example of how to set things right.

5. **Choose your new milk.** One of the easiest steps toward a vegan diet is to change from dairy to nondairy milk (see page 217). You might want to have a "milk sampling," akin to a wine tasting, to discover which milk suits you. There are more choices than ever before: hemp seed milk, almond milk, sunflower milk, soy milk, rice milk, and combinations like rice-soy, cashew-hazelnut, or almond-coconut. A milk tasting could be a family event, or a theme for a get-together with friends.

You could arrange a blind taste test or simply sip each kind of milk in turn. Many vegans use different milks for different recipes and different purposes. And even among soy milks there are many choices: original or unsweetened, vanilla, chocolate, and refrigerated or aseptic boxes (which have a longer shelf life and do not need to be refrigerated).

VEGANS OVER 50 TELL THEIR STORIES

Never Too Late to Change the World: Why I Became Vegetarian at Age 86 | Sherrey Reim Glickman*

Sherrey's story: Born in 1924 into a Jewish immigrant household in Brooklyn, I was raised on chicken soup, meat loaf, gefilte fish, hamburgers, hot dogs, and steak. I loved them all, never questioning what the source of my food was. Everyone I knew lived and ate the same way. Thanksgiving was for eating turkey. Passover was for eating chicken or pot roast. Factory farming hadn't yet boomed. Perhaps animals were treated better, but then again, they were still slaughtered for food. And who even thought about that, anyway? Eating meat was the norm of the day.

When I got married to George, I was eighteen. I continued to cook as my mother had, except I added more vegetables to our diet. George was a very open-minded, progressive guy, who always questioned assumptions. He marched with Martin Luther King, Jr., an experience that forever changed him. He was the kind of partner who encouraged me to follow my dreams. He was not the sort of man who would be embarrassed by a working wife—though that was the thinking of many at that time. As a

---

* This first-person story by Sherrey Reim Glickman is adapted from what first appeared in the online magazine Our Hen House (OurHenHouse.org), a nonprofit multimedia hub of opportunities to change the world for animals. Sherrey's granddaughter, Jasmin Singer, and Mariann Sullivan, cofounders of Our Hen House are referred to in the piece.

result, I led a happy, fulfilled life. The reason I bring this up is, had we known about the exploitation of animals then, and about veganism (a word that was not even coined yet), George would have become a vegan and embraced animal rights activism. I'm sure of it. Too bad we didn't know about that lifestyle. Maybe he would have lived longer. My George died way too young, of a fast and furious cancer that took his life in a matter of months.

My second husband, Murray, loved animals. He took more pleasure in talking about his dog than about his children. . . . Had Murray been alive when *Our Hen House* started, he would have been an activist for the cause.

So how did I change, and why? How did I become who I am, instead of who I was?

I had always been an activist for women's rights. I lived life as a woman who moved to the beat of her own drum. It seems like a natural extension that animal rights came next.

When my darling granddaughter Jasmin went to work for Farm Sanctuary, I became a little involved. I bought Gene Baur's book *Changing Hearts and Minds About Animals and Food,* and I went to Princeton to hear his lecture. I attended the NYC Walk for Farm Animals, and marveled at what a movement this cause had become. I attended meetings and workshops where they showed films documenting how animals were being abused. These films were very graphic, and not easy to swallow. I did not realize how much I was being affected.

I shared my feelings with my friends. Their reactions were mostly sympathetic; they realized that animals were not treated humanely. One of my friends decided to become a vegetarian. The others told me it was too late to change their eating habits. I had not yet declared myself a vegetarian, although I was eating differently and didn't realize it. When I joined my family at restaurants, I discovered how tasty vegan food is.

Then, when I read Mariann's letter to the editor in *The New York Times Magazine*, regarding how deeply we as a culture are impacted by the massive denial our society has when it comes to consuming animal products—consuming death, really—it had a profound effect on me. That letter was, I see now, my last straw, the final step in making a decision regarding the path I must take. I declared myself a vegetarian, putting an important label on a behavior I realized I had already adopted. I now knew, without any doubt, why I could no longer eat meat. It was a declaration for my future, and for the future of the planet. Meat made me sick. At long last, there was simply no way I could continue to support the cruelty of animal production. The world evolves, and so do we.

So who am I at this point of my life? I was eighty-six when I made such dramatic changes. I no longer join my friends for lunch, because even the smell of meat cooking makes me ill—and not just physically.

I am now an eighty-eight-year-old dame living in a vegan home. My daughter cooks colorful, healthy, decadent, delicious meals for me. I eat better than I ever have before. I am happy to have changed the way I eat, and the way I think. I am angry that society accepts the way we treat our animals, and I will continue to espouse the rights of animals. I like who I am now!

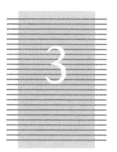

WHY VEGAN?
VEGANISM IS A SIMPLE AND EFFECTIVE RESPONSE TO A SERIES OF COMPLEX CONTEMPORARY ISSUES

VEGANISM IS FAR more than a personal food choice. It is a simple and effective response to a series of complex contemporary issues affecting animals, personal health, and the environment.

Most of us shy away from knowing the full story of where our food comes from, and it's true that the information presented in this chapter is very sad. But as we mature we are asked to live with our eyes and hearts wide open. We are old enough and, having seen our share of tragedies over the decades, able to handle the information about why vegan.

We who are over fifty have learned that our capacity to recover from bad news is stronger than we thought it was. In fact, we've learned that grief is endurable; it is part of living. Because we've had these experiences in living, we are prepared to learn about what is happening to animals and our planet and not turn away from it.

. . .

THE VEGAN ANSWER TO SOME PRESSING CONCERNS

Consider the challenges of our contemporary world:

- heart disease, diabetes, cancer, and other health problems
- shrinking polar ice caps, destruction of rainforests, ozone depletion, and other effects associated with climate change
- environmental effects of factory farms and feedlots—the sewage waste and toxic fumes they produce and their dependence on fossil fuels—as well as the treatment of animals
- the depletion of fresh water in aquifers and overused rivers, and the "desertification" of our oceans, decline of coral reefs, and disruption to maritime ecosystems
- the extinction of fish species and land animals at record numbers
- violence as a way of life

Choosing a vegan lifestyle provides a simple and effective response to these complex issues. It is one of the easiest ways we know to improve our own health while also lessening the burden of our choices on animals and the environment.

ANIMAL AGRICULTURE AND THE ENVIRONMENT

In *Diet for a Small Planet*, Dr. Frances Moore Lappé referred to beef production as a "protein factory in reverse." What she meant was that we feed huge amounts of protein in the form of grain and soybeans to cattle in order to produce relatively small amounts of beef. The output—the protein in the beef—is far smaller than the input—the protein in the corn and soybeans.

Dr. Lappé suggested that the average steer reduces 16 pounds of soybeans and grains to a single pound of meat. Where do the other 15 pounds go? They are used by the animal for energy production or for growth of some part of the body that we don't eat, or it is lost in manure.

The actual numbers are debated and they differ according to type of animal and the type of food the animal consumes. But while the numbers may vary, the basic concept remains true: When we feed grain and soybeans to animals to produce meat, milk, and eggs, much of the protein and energy are lost. Loss of energy and protein isn't just wasteful, it is also devastating to the environment. This is because, if we got our protein directly from grains and beans, we would not need to grow nearly so much of them. We would need less farmland, less water, and smaller amounts of fossil fuels.

Land is a big issue, according to the Food and Agricultural Organization (FAO) of the United Nations, which has calculated that nearly a third of the earth's land surface is devoted to production of animals for food, when we take into consideration land used for grazing and for growing feed for those animals. And we can expect to need much more in the future. As the population grows and animal food consumption continues, global production of meat is expected to double by the year 2050.

The FAO says that, today, 70 percent of land in the Amazon that was once rainforest has been cleared to graze cattle or to produce soybeans for cattle feed. If we ate soybeans (and other beans and grains) directly we wouldn't need nearly as much land and could leave the rainforest alone. The rainforest canopy is important for clearance of the carbon dioxide that contributes to global warming, so its loss can have far-reaching effects on the health of the planet. Loss of rainforest also means loss of habitat for tropical species.

The incredible inefficiency of meat and dairy production means that it wastes other resources as well. It takes far more water to produce protein from cows, pigs, and chickens than we would need if we simply ate grains and beans. For example, the FAO reports that it can take 990 liters of water just to produce 1 liter of cow's milk.[1] Most of this water isn't being fed directly to the cow. It's being used to irrigate crops for the cow to eat. In turn, waste from animals along with fertilizers and pesticides used to grow their food contributes to water pollution. Sediment from eroded pastures also contributions to pollution.

The FAO points to the global livestock industry as probably "the largest sectoral source of water pollution." Animal agriculture also produces massive amounts of methane, which contributes to global warming. As much as 18 percent of global greenhouse gas emissions are attributable to animal farming. Animals also produce massive amounts of manure full of nitrogen, phosphorous and potassium, along with drug residues, heavy metals, and pathogens.[2] As much as 18 percent of global greenhouse gas emissions are attributable to animal farming.

Whether raised in factory farms or family farms, the animals still produce manure, nitrous oxide, methane, and urine. There is nothing magical about raising animals in smaller numbers. According to the USDA, each lactating dairy cow produces about 150 pounds of manure a day, each "dry" cow about 83 pounds per day, or about 25 tons of manure annually.[3] And the Environmental Protection Agency reports that a broiler chicken produces 11 pounds of manure during a short lifetime of seven weeks, while each hog excretes 1,200 pounds of manure yearly.[4] Runoff from animal agriculture is seeping into our groundwater, polluting our air, and causing a stench that the animals and their human neighbors must live with every day.

When you consider the effects of all these inputs and outputs, it becomes clear that production of animal food is one big vicious cycle that takes a tremendous toll on the health of our planet. Animal agriculture gobbles up land as we grow huge amounts of crops for the production of small amounts of animal food—the protein factory in reverse. The animals produce gases that contribute to global warming, but the rainforest—which could help to counter the effects of those gases—has shrunk because we've cleared it to grow food for the animals. Crops for animals need huge amounts of water; in turn, the excrement resulting from meat production causes water pollution, further shrinking supplies of this precious resource.

There is always a cost to food production. Growing plant food impacts the environment, too. But we have to eat. And we can reduce our burden on the planet by eating the foods that take less land, water, and fuel and that produce less pollution. We do this by adopting a diet based on plant foods.

THE HUNGER CONNECTION

MORE THAN 870 MILLION of the world's people have insufficient food, according to the UN World Food Programme's Hunger Statistics.[5] It's a complex problem that has far more to do with politics and poverty than with food availability. If we could get food to the world's hungry, we could feed them.

According to Walden Bello, former CEO of the Institute for Food and Development Policy, "The fact is that there is enough food in the world for everyone. But tragically, much of the world's food and land resources are tied up producing beef and other livestock-food for the well-off, while millions of children and adults suffer from malnutrition and starvation."[6]

That may change, though, as the world's population grows and our resources shrink. We're going to have to get much more efficient if we want to feed a growing hungry planet. Sociobiologist Edward O. Wilson, PhD, of Harvard University, estimates that the planet can support between 9 and 10 billion people if we are all vegetarian. Right now, the earth's population stands at more than 7 billion and we can expect to reach 9 billion by the year 2044.[7]

OUR VEGAN LIVES

Why and How We Talk About the Lives of Animals

Carol: For some readers, our discussion of the lives of farmed animals may feel as though we have entered a terrain with language that carries heightened emotion. "What's going on?" you might wonder. In the mainstream press, veganism is often portrayed mainly as a healthy, plant-based way of living. But many vegans chose this way of living precisely because they did not want meals based on animals' deaths. Such a realization has been called by philosopher Mary Midgley a "gestalt shift." (Gestalt means "whole" or "pattern.") Midgley explains it this way: "The symbolism of meat-eating is never neutral. To himself, the meat-eater seems to be eating life. To the vegetarian, he seems to be eating death. There is a kind of gestalt-shift between the two positions which makes it hard to change, and hard to raise questions on the matter at all without becoming embattled."[8] In my own life, with just one bite, I shifted from seeing myself as eating life to eating death.

While traveling on an airplane once, I was seated next to a child psychologist. We had already engaged in a long, relaxed conversation about his profession and his work with troubled, gifted children. When my vegan meal was delivered to my seat, this prompted a discussion. He admitted knowing that meat eating was unethical, but still persisting in his ways. Because we had already explored many topics, I felt comfortable turning to him and asking what this conflict felt like: "What happens, then, when you sit down to eat meat?"

"I have a hole in my conscience," he said.

I thought about that, a compelling and honest answer. But I was troubled. "But our entire culture says it's okay," I responded.

He replied: "Well, we've got a collective hole in our conscience."

It may help to consider our discussion of farmed animals as our attempt to repair the hole in our conscience.

Patti: I became an activist because I believe that the animals who have no voice can use my big mouth. When I see the way we treat animals raised for food—on the websites of PETA, Mercy for Animals, United Poultry Concerns, Friends of Animals, Compassion over Killing, Animal Place—I cannot sit by and pretend I have nothing to do with that abuse. Although he was referring to people when he wrote them, when I read the words of Elie Weisel—"We must take sides. Neutrality helps the oppressor, never the victim. Silence encourages the tormentor, never the tormented."—I knew that I had to get involved to help stop the needless violence and unnecessary killing of innocent animals.

Whenever I think of a way to spread the word about veganism, I try my best to take advantage of the opportunity to do so. Sometimes it is as simple as wearing a T-shirt showing a picture of a cow with the caption "Someone, not something." Other times, it means writing letters to a newspaper in response to an article about heart disease, climate change, or the circus or the rodeo that is in the news. I attend as many conferences as I can to hear from experts in health, the environment, and animal issues, and I write a monthly newsletter that is sent by e-mail to local members of the Marin Vegetarian Education Group.

Because I am active in the study and practice of Buddhism, I joined with others in the Dharma community to create Dharma Voices for Animals (dharmavoicesforanimals.org). We are working to bring awareness of the suffering of animals to everyone in that community. (Dharma refers to the teachings of the Buddha.) Nonharming is a basic tenet of Buddhism, and yet so many people do not know about the harm we cause to animals when our food choices are rooted in habit and not awareness. So many people never learned about the damage we do when we eat the way we were taught to as children.

By talking about what animals experience, I am hoping to change habit into awareness.

Ginny: Because I'm a dietitian, and it's my job to talk about the health impacts of food choices, people are often surprised to learn that I went vegan for the animals. I was, in fact, a dietitian for quite a few years before I adopted a vegan diet. I was also one of those people whose cholesterol, blood pressure, and weight all stayed low no matter how many ice-cream sundaes I ate. So I didn't feel much motivation to change my diet for my health.

I used to think that how we eat is all about meeting nutrient needs and protecting ourselves from chronic disease. And those are still driving forces behind the kind of advice I give about nutrition and the type of food choices I make for myself. But if we stop at those concerns—as important as they are—it's a pretty limited and narrow way of looking at food choices. Food choices have such far-reaching impacts. As a nutrition professional, I feel obligated to share information that acknowledges the impacts, not just on health, but on the lives of animals and the environment, too.

THE LIVES OF FARMED ANIMALS

Current agricultural processes are committed to producing animal protein quickly and cheaply. Industry's interest is not in the lives of individual animals; rather, it is focused on maximizing profit. The agricultural industry refers to current farming techniques as concentrated animal feeding operations, or CAFOs. Critics note that farms have turned into animal factories, giving rise to the term *factory farm*.

It's a vast system, resulting in the death of 10 billion animals every year in the United States alone. It's hard to wrap your mind around those numbers. We can't really imagine that many animals, let alone hold that much suffering in our heart. So we tune out. But when we hear stories about individual animals, we're reminded that each is a living, breathing creature who desires life and freedom. For example, take the story about a cow who came to be called Cinci Freedom. In the winter of 2002, she jumped a 6-foot fence to escape a Cincinnati meatpacking plant. For eleven days, despite attempts to capture her, she ran free in a city park where she eluded the SPCA officials. Her run for freedom garnered more and more attention around the world.

Cincinnati's mayor, Charlie Luken, pledged to give her a key to the city. Finally, she was captured.

People had become emotionally attached to the cow, and, clearly, she was not going to be returned to the slaughterhouse to be killed. Artist Peter Max offered some of his artwork to ensure that she would be able to live in freedom.

She was indeed given the key to the city and then transported to Farm Sanctuary, a haven for rescued farmed animals in upstate New York. Before heading to her new home, she was marched through the city of Cincinnati in a parade celebrating the start of baseball season. Those who celebrated her freedom applauded the rescued cow and then headed to the ballpark to eat hot dogs and hamburgers made from cows who didn't manage to escape the slaughterhouse. Yet, each of the cows who died to produce those ballpark snacks was as deserving of life and humane treatment as Cinci Freedom.

If you find yourself going numb when you read about enormous numbers of animals who suffer and die on factory farms, then hold just one animal—one like Cinci Freedom—in your heart. Every time you pass up meat, milk, and eggs, you are saying no to the abuse of an individual animal who would run from the slaughterhouse if she could.

The Lives of Pigs on Factory Farms

Have you seen the T-shirt with a picture of a pig on it that says, "No, I don't have any spare ribs."?

More than 100 million pigs are killed for food every year in the United States, and more than 60 million live in factory farms today. Worldwide the numbers are even more staggering.

Like chickens, turkeys, and cows, every pig has an individual personality and a will to live as strong as any human's. Each of those 100 million pigs is an intelligent, friendly, and curious animal. When able to, pigs will come to greet a human friend and follow her around as a dog might. Pigs love belly rubs and like to take mud baths to cool off because they don't have sweat glands.

Despite this, female pigs raised for food spend most of their lives in gestation crates, metal crates that are too small for the pig to even turn around. A few days before giving birth, they are moved to farrowing crates from which they cannot cuddle or touch or build nests for their offspring. The sow still cannot turn around. For ten days, the piglets nurse through metal bars. Then, they are taken away from their mothers, castrated, have their tails cut off without anesthesia, and raised for meat. The mothers are again impregnated and moved back into a gestation crate. The cycle of cruelty continues.

Chickens and Other Birds Raised for Meat

Efficiency on factory farms depends on animals who grow quickly. Birds raised for meat are bred to grow so quickly that they suffer leg deformities, heart attacks, and other organ failure. As many as 26 percent of chickens raised for meat are severely crippled and 90 percent cannot walk normally by the time they reach slaughter weight. This lameness is so prevalent and painful that some breeds of chickens will routinely choose food that has painkillers added to it over regular feed.

In the slaughterhouse, the six-week-old chickens are quickly killed and then dropped into scalding tanks. If the blade misses, chickens may still be alive when they land in those tanks of boiling water. According to government statistics, as many as a million birds may die this way every year. A Tyson slaughterhouse worker reported, "They often come out the other end with broken bones and disfigured and missing body parts because they've struggled so much in the tank."[9]

Consider the Animal in "Feminized Protein"

In her book *The Sexual Politics of Meat*, Carol coined the term *feminized protein* to describe foods that are the products of female reproduction— eggs and milk. Although these animals eventually go to slaughter just like those raised for meat, they first spend lives of misery on farms.

Egg-Laying Hens

Life for these animals begins in the hatchery. This is true for factory farmed birds as well as so called "humanely" raised birds and even for backyard chickens. Within minutes of hatching, male chicks (who have no value in egg production) are tossed into a pile to be suffocated in plastic bags or thrown into a disposal unit, a bigger version of the one you might have in your kitchen sink, to be ground up alive. Sometimes they are just left to die in Dumpsters, and in some facilities, they are gassed. When people order baby chicks for their home chicken coops, sometimes the males are used as "packing material," and added to the box of female chicks to insulate them as they travel through the mail.

And yet, being killed on your first day alive might be a better fate than what awaits the female chicks. The life of a "laying hen" is one of confinement, mutilation, and depletion. Most hens are packed into cages so small the birds cannot spread their wings. The animals' beaks are seared off—this is called debeaking—without anesthesia to keep birds from pecking one another in confined quarters. Their feet frequently become deformed from standing in wire enclosures day after day and sometimes wrap around and fuse to the wires. In some facilities, excrement from the birds in the higher tiers falls onto the birds below.

In nature, chickens love to take dust baths, develop relationships with one another and establish pecking orders, bask in the sun, roost in trees, prepare nests, and protect their offspring with tender dedication. People who share their lives with chickens know that they are personable, friendly, affectionate companions. But factory farms are structured to thwart their chickenness. Birds are denied the ability to exercise most of their natural behaviors because egg production and profit are the only priorities in egg laying facilities.

"Free-range" or "cage-free" chickens also live short, sad lives. They are usually kept by the thousands in huge warehouses, with access through one small door to a tiny patch of outdoor space. In fact, most of these "free-range" chickens never see daylight. And like caged chickens, they have their beaks seared off and their brothers are all killed at the hatchery. All egg-laying hens are sent to slaughter when their egg production falls off. There is cruelty in eggs, no matter where they come from and how they are raised.

Dairy Cows and Veal Calves

A dairy cow is impregnated every year because only cows who have given birth can produce milk. Within twenty-four hours of birth, her baby is taken away from her. Her milk is for humans, after all, not for raising her own babies. Mother cows grieve for their young. Meanwhile, female calves are often raised in isolation until they are old enough to start producing milk. The males are also raised in isolation for a few short, sad months, and then they are killed for veal. The life of a dairy cow is an endless cycle of misery; she suffers from an exhausting life of milk production. For nine months of every year, she will be both pregnant and lactating. Her udders often become engorged and infected. Under natural circumstances, a dairy cow could live for twenty years. But by the age of four, the average dairy cow is depleted and her milk production declines. She is sent to slaughter, sometimes so weakened at this point that she becomes a "downer cow," unable to even walk off the truck to slaughter.

Her life might be even shorter if she lives on an organic dairy farm. If she develops mastitis or any other infection, she can't be treated with antibiotics on these farms and so will be killed for meat.

Because plant foods can provide abundant calcium, along with many other nutrients important for bone health, we have no need for these products of misery in our diets. And with a growing selection of vegan cheeses and milks on the market, it's increasingly easy to ditch dairy.

HOW TO GIVE UP CHEESE

▶ Learn the truth about cows, calves, and the dairy industry. When you are educated about the inherent violence of repeated artificial insemination, the wrenching sadness of calves crying for their mothers, the loss the mother feels after carrying her young for nine months, and the unconscionable profits the dairy industry makes from the exploitation of gentle cows and their slaughter, you will be motivated to find alternatives to dairy cheese.

▶ Discover nondairy cheeses. Jo Stepaniak wrote the first bible of homemade nondairy cheeses, *The Ultimate UnCheese Cookbook.* Subsequently, Miyoko Schinner wrote a remarkable book about making cultured nondairy cheeses, *Artisan Vegan Cheese.* See pages 221–225 in our book for a few recipes for vegan cheese and then seek out those two definitive books for more. If you don't like to cook, look for Daiya cheese, a tapioca-based nondairy cheese found in most natural foods stores. Other wonderful vegan cheeses include Teese, Dr. Cow, Vegan Gourmet, and Go Veggie!

▶ Try nutritional yeast. Nutritional yeast (not yeast for bread baking) is a wonderful condiment. It's available as flakes or powder and can be sprinkled on popcorn, soup, salads, and other dishes to add a hint of cheeselike flavor. Carol ran into a man in the supermarket who was buying 2 tablespoons for a recipe. She explained why he might want to buy at least a cup or two. Keep it handy in a jar in your kitchen and you will find that adding it to many different foods helps to curb your cheese craving.

▶ Discover umami. In addition to our taste buds for salty, sweet, bitter, and sour flavors, we also have receptors for umami, a savory aspect of some foods, which was discovered in Japan more than one hundred years ago. Cheese is especially notable for umami, but so are many plant foods. If you find yourself craving cheese, try adding more umami-rich plant foods and ingredients to your menus. The best sources of umami include:

- *Fermented foods:* wine, tamari (soy sauce), sauerkraut, tempeh (a savory "patty" made from fermented soybeans and sometimes also grains), and miso. Miso is a salty, fermented soybean paste that captures the essence of Japanese cooking. It comes in different colors—white, red, and yellow—and some are somewhat sweeter than others. It's used extensively in vegan broths, soups, sauces, and for making homemade vegan cheeses.
- *Sea vegetables*, often referred to as seaweed because they grow wild in the ocean, include nori, kombu, dulse, arame, and kelp, and play a big role in Japanese cooking. They are usually sold dried and then can be added to soups or used to make vegetarian sushi.
- *Balsamic vinegar*
- *Ume plum vinegar* is made from the pickling brine from umeboshi plums. Unlike other vinegars, it's high in salt, so use it sparingly. Its umami-laden flavor means a few drops go a long way.
- *Marmite*, a thick, yeast-based spread. It's a very salty condiment so a little goes a long way. It's an especially umami-rich food. Some people swear by Marmite on sandwiches, especially in Great Britain and Australia.
- *Ripe tomatoes and concentrated tomato products*, such as sun-dried tomatoes, tomato paste, and ketchup
- *Nutritional yeast* (see above)
- *Mushrooms*, including dried mushrooms
- *Olives*
- *Roasting, caramelizing, browning and grilling* all boost compounds that contribute to umami, making foods more umami-rich.

▶ Just say no. You can always say, "No cheese, please," when ordering a burrito, pizza, salad, wrap, or sandwich. Ask to substitute avocado at Subway or Taco Bell. Delis will often substitute hummus for cheese. (By the way, when having your picture taken, saying "vegan" produces the same smile as saying "cheese.")

WHAT ABOUT LOCAVORE, ORGANIC MEAT, AND HUMANE SLAUGHTER?

Such phrases as *humanely raised, happy meat, organically raised, free-range, grown locally, cage-free, family farms,* and other expressions of alternatives to factory farms would be terrific if only their feel-good message actually meant something. Unfortunately, there are precious few laws to define what any of these terms means.

Animals raised with any of those labels are still bred the same, born the same, removed from their mothers, subjected to mutilation, and then slaughtered at the same slaughterhouses where the factory farmed animals are killed.

People who say, "I only eat humanely raised meat," may not realize that there is really no such thing. After all, if someone treated their puppy well for a few months and then killed him, you probably wouldn't refer to that person as humane. *Humane* labels may ease the meat eater's conscience, but they are deceptive. They don't help animals and they often have the same damaging effects on the environment. If you want to make a difference to animals and the earth, be kind to your body, and be at peace with your conscience, the only real choice is to go vegan.

Counting Animals

Each vegetarian saves about 30 land animals, 225 fish, and 151 shellfish every year, according to CountingAnimals.com. This website, "a place for people who love animals and numbers," uses a careful formula for its calculations. It includes not only the animals people eat, but also the sea animals killed as "by-catch" when the fishing industry uses enormous nets and huge ships to catch targeted species.

The founder of Counting Animals, Harish, says, "We have always known that billions of animals are slaughtered for our food. What surprised me was the pre-slaughter mortality rate caused by the harsh conditions in which they are raised. The animals experience such severe physical breakdown during their short lives that hundreds of millions of them suffer to death even before they reach the moment of slaughter."[10]

We cannot live five decades or more without seeing that every action has a consequence. Our food choices affect real animals. While many injustices are beyond the scope of our influence, the injustice to farmed animals is very much ours to end.

HEALTH ISSUES

Eating plant foods helps us in two different and potentially powerful ways. First, removing animal foods from your diet automatically eliminates cholesterol (it's never found in plants) and will greatly reduce your intake of saturated fats. Replacing these saturated fats with fiber-rich carbohydrates and fats from plant foods causes direct (and sometimes dramatic) reductions in blood cholesterol levels. It prevents processes that lead to clogged arteries and heart disease. Saturated fat may be linked to other chronic diseases, too, such as cancer and Alzheimer's disease.

But vegan diets aren't just about what we don't eat. Plants are rich in fiber, which protects intestinal health, moderates blood glucose levels, and may reduce risk for heart disease and some types of cancer. Plants also provide thousands of chemicals—phytochemicals—that act in myriad ways to protect our health. These are the nonnutrient compounds that appear to have all kinds of important health benefits. Some step in to counter processes leading to cancer, while others protect the health of the arteries. Certain phytochemicals could protect the health of your brain and slow aging in the layers of your skin.

Plants are packed with nutrients, too. Some nutrients, such as potassium, are often more abundant in vegetarian and vegan diets. Potassium is needed for healthy bones and to keep blood pressure in check. Vegans also consume more folate, a B vitamin needed for a healthy heart, and vitamin C, important for the health of your immune system.

Not surprisingly, people who eat plant-based diets have lower risks for heart disease, diabetes, and some cancers. Vegans tend to have lower cholesterol levels, often even compared to those eating other types of vegetarian diets. Although researchers aren't quite sure why, vegans often have lower blood pressures. And there is evidence to suggest that vegans have a lower body weight and less diabetes. Vegan diets have also been used with great success to treat people who have chronic diseases, such as diabetes and heart disease.

Maybe we can't say with certainty that you have to be 100 percent vegan to enjoy all of these health perks. Neither are we saying that a vegan diet will guarantee perfect health. For one thing, diet is only one part of a health-promoting lifestyle that also includes exercise, stress management, positive social interaction, and smoking cessation. But when you factor in the benefits to animals and the environment, then it makes sense to adopt a vegan diet and enjoy the health benefits it can bring. We'll talk much more about health benefits of plant foods, as well as how to make your vegan diet as health-promoting as possible, in chapters 5 and 6.

VEGANISM IS KINDNESS IN ACTION

The problems in the world today need our wisdom and our compassion. And there is no better place to begin to exercise these qualities than in our kitchens. Once we step out of our role as consumers in the system that breeds, confines, mutilates, and kills animals, we can begin to nurture that warm connection to the other beings with whom we share our planet.

"Being vegan has changed my life for the better in so many ways. I began to bring other aspects of my life into harmony with my new values, and returned to meditating every day. I'm a clinical psychologist by profession. And my specialty most of my career has been trauma and

its lasting effects on its victims as well as those exposed to the traumas of others, such as witnessing domestic violence. When we participate even indirectly in the terror and painful deaths of animals for our appetites, we bear some of that trauma and it damages us psychologically." — SHIELAGH (62)

You don't have to become an activist, holding signs at protest marches (although some of us choose that route). You merely have to acknowledge that living beings are hurt when we choose to eat their body or their bodily secretions, and then act in a way that no longer hurts these beings.

As vegan consumers we are conscious of the impact of each purchase on other beings. As animal lovers we are aware of the lives and deaths of cows, pigs, chickens, turkeys, goats, lambs, and sheep when we look at a menu, ingredient list, or clothing label (see "Beyond Food Choices"). We make choices that matter to these beings. We try our best to live with conscious awareness and thoughtfulness. We use our intention to be kind to other beings to bring about the world that we hope to create.

"Veganism is the touchstone of my life. As I wrote recently on Our Hen House, it's not . . . a dietary preference or even a 'social philosophy.' For me, it is a fundamental moral imperative, one that drives my life, based in my deepest beliefs about my role in the world and my relationships with its other inhabitants. Veganism is at the core of the way I live. It is always there, and I have come to it through both thought and emotion. It makes the world work for me." —MARIANN (63)

BEYOND FOOD CHOICES

AS YOU MOVE TOWARD veganism, you will probably become aware of other ways animals are used and abused. Because our focus is on kindness, and not only personal health, vegans pay attention to the needless suffering animals endure in entertainment, clothing, laboratories, hunting, and other industries.

As vegans, we seek out entertainment that doesn't exploit animals. We might choose Cirque de Soleil rather than a circus that uses trained elephants and lions. We look for household products and personal care products that are free of animal ingredients and haven't been tested on animals. An easy way to do this is by looking for "bunny" logos on products—either a leaping bunny or bunny ears to signify that the product is cruelty-free. You can even download smart phone apps, such as "Be Nice to Bunnies," that will help you shop.

Finally, vegans have fun building new cruelty-free wardrobes, since leather, fur, feathers, silk, and wool are all produced at the expense of animal suffering and death. We opt for cotton, linen, and hemp, as well as newer fibers made from bamboo and even soy, along with fun synthetics, such as pleather.

While treatment of animals for nonfood purposes is beyond the scope of this book, we can recommend a few good books that will help you learn more about these issues:

Why Animals Matter by Erin E. Williams and Margo DeMello
Bleating Hearts: The Hidden World of Animal Suffering by Mark Hawthorne
The World Peace Diet by Will Tuttle, PhD

When we are in the second half of our life, through veganism we can discover ways of connecting or reconnecting to the entire world, to make a difference with every meal, to express our beliefs through our actions.

"During the entire time, I have felt at peace with animals and the environment—and still do. Being vegan relates to my social justice focus in life. I am still active in animal rights and work with two animal rescue organizations." —LORI (60)

We may miss some of the central roles we once played as parents or as important cogs in the wheels of a working life. But now we see that the role we are called to as a steward of our planet, a protector of the defenseless, an advocate for wise, health supporting choices can be one of the most important and most effective (and delicious) roles of our lifetime. We have seen enough needless violence in our lives and we know the value of choosing another way.

We don't need Congress to change the animal protection laws (though that would be ideal, as farmed animals are excluded from many of them, and birds are exempt from the few laws animals do have to protect them). We don't need anybody's permission to act. We simply stop eating animals and products made from animals and start eating plants.

VEGANS OVER 50 TELL THEIR STORIES:

"You Can Add Compassion to the World" | Marc Bekoff

Marc's story: Marc Bekoff is professor emeritus of ecology and evolutionary biology at the University of Colorado, Boulder. Marc's specialty is cognitive ethology—the study of animal minds. Marc explains that people come to this area of study from many different angles. He comes to it from an ethological approach; that is, watching the animals, trying to understand why their brains and minds evolved the way they did. He says this is a naturalist approach. "We ask questions, such as, 'What do they know?,' 'What do they feel?,' 'Are they moral beings?'" Marc points out that many animals have highly evolved moral sentiments. For him, the bottom line is to show that they are not just objects or machines; they are *whos*, not *whats*.

His other specialty is behavioral ecology: how environmental variables influence behavior. "Animals show variability in behavior and social organization, so talking about '*the* coyote' or '*the* wolf,' is misleading. It is a very simplistic attitude that allows in some ways for exploitation. When people say, 'Coyotes do this, so we can do this to them,' this is an error: in fact, coyotes show great variation and flexibility in behavior. This ties in with animal welfare, compassionate conservation treating animals as individuals who have a life. 'I am a coyote, but I may not behave like all other coyotes.' It is a very powerful move to get people to think about animals as individuals."

Marc has published more than twenty-two books; his most recent ones include scholarly texts on cognitive ethology and behavioral ecology, *Wild Justice: The Moral Lives of Animals* and *Compassionate Conservation*.

Marc's work in cognitive ethology has led him directly to confront the raising and slaughtering of animals for food. He says the issue isn't *what* we eat but *who* we eat. He explains, "Cognitive ethology and other current studies are showing that animals are individuals. They are feeling and sentient beings, who also want what we want, which is to live in peace and safety. Exploiting animals for food or for clothes and entertainment is a form of violence. People don't like to think about it that way, but it is sanctioned violence. It is wrong on a lot of accounts. It is wrong because most of us, not all of us, have non-animal alternatives. We have sufficient alternatives to exploiting animals and abusing them. What science is showing us, though we have known this forever, is that animals care about what is happening to them, and we should treat them with respect and dignity, that they have a point of view about what happens to them and to their family and friends."

Two recent developments in meat production have received

Marc's attention: First, Temple Grandin's work to try to make slaughterhouses less stressful for animals as they walk up what she calls the "Stairway to Heaven" as they are on the way to being killed. Second, the emergence of organic and local farmers with their assertions that their animals are "happy" before slaughter.

Marc asks, "Would you put your dog in a factory farm or on a 'happy farm'?"

Marc has challenged Grandin: "You say you understand these animals; so why aren't you working to protect them and save them so they won't be killed?" He also notes that in addition to her book earnings, Grandin receives income from meat companies she defends.

To be fair, Marc says, "She may be responsible for making 0.001 percent of their lives better, but *better* doesn't mean a good life. These animals are suffering in the slaughterhouse. You can't control it all: they hear the other animals, they see them, they smell them, and they are picking up their pain, suffering, and death.

"Temple may be providing a better life, but it surely isn't close to a good life. A Cadillac may get better mileage than a Hummer, but it isn't good mileage." He continues, "No animal who winds up in the factory farm production line has a good or even moderately good life, one that we would allow our dogs or cats to experience. In fact, their lives are marked by constant fear, terror, and anxiety. A 'better' life on a factory farm isn't close to being marginally 'good.'"

Marc is also concerned about what he calls the "born again carnivory" that he finds justifying "happy farms." In an article for the *Atlantic*, entitled "Dead Cow Walking: The Case Against Born-Again Carnivorism," he wrote, "Cows, for example, are very intelligent. They worry over what they don't understand and have been shown to experience 'eureka' moments when they solve a puzzle, such as when they figure out how to open a particularly difficult gate. Cows communicate by staring, and it's likely that we don't fully understand their very subtle forms of communication. They also form close and enduring relationships with family members and friends and don't like to have their families and social networks disrupted. Chickens are also emotional beings, and detailed scientific research has shown that they empathize with the pain of other chickens."

He says that from an ethical point of view it is wrong to bring an animal into the world who you know you will kill for a meal you don't need. From a sentience point of view, the animals are instruments. You are raising this animal for your own needs. "We are choosing to slaughter sentience. It's a major double cross, you bring a cow into the world and treat them well and then slit their throat."

The "happy animal" argument proposes that by raising contented animals and then killing them separated from the other animals on the farm (often the same slaughterhouses as factory-farmed animals), they are providing everything the animal needs. The problem with this argument, Marc points out, is that it looks at each animal only in relationship to humans and not to the other animals with whom they are living. "Whether the other animals know that their friend was killed or just went off to the movie, they still miss that animal. Farmers are taking friends from one another; they are breaking up social groups. We all know how animals miss one another."

Marc retired from teaching at the University of Colorado in 2006, but he is busier than ever. While Boulder continues to be his home, he travels around the world lecturing on "animal minds." When people tell Marc they love animals and then harm them (through "happy farms" or in other ways), he tells them, "I'm glad you don't love me."

For many years, Marc was 99.9 percent vegan; for the past seven years he has been 100 percent vegan. His advice for becoming a vegan is "Do it slowly. Don't go 'cold tofu.' Start cutting back slowly. Focus on making sure you get the nutrients you need. Monitor how you feel." He urges people to stop the distancing devices that protect their eating habits. He suggests it is not a bacon, lettuce, and tomato sandwich but a "Babe, lettuce, and tomato sandwich."

Most important, "Factor in the notion of compassion. By becoming vegan, you are making a great contribution to the world: you will see you really don't need to have animals in your diet. You are adding compassion to the world."

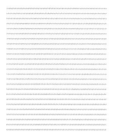

PART TWO

NUTRITION FOR THE 50+ BODY

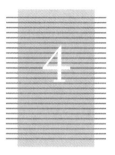

WHY AND HOW WE AGE

FROM THE MOMENT we're born our bodies are changing. We grow and then go through a process of sexual maturation. One theory is that aging begins right after puberty.

Some of the age-related changes do begin to look and feel more obvious by our fifties, though. And many of them are inevitable. But while we can't stop the clock, there is no doubt that we can slow things down.

It's true that there is a genetic component to aging and longevity. Researchers who study the long-lived Okinawan population have identified "human longevity genes" that may reduce risk for some chronic diseases.[1] But while genetics may explain as much as one third of longevity, most of *how* we age is under the influence of other factors, including diet and lifestyle.

We can protect our skin, bones, and muscles through the years and it's never too late to start doing so. We can also prevent many of the chronic diseases that we often associate with aging. A healthy vegan diet can be a powerful prescription for staying well.

In this chapter we'll look at what happens to men and women as they enter the second half of life. In chapters 5 and 6 we'll see how diet affects these processes and also how it counters some of the chronic diseases that are so prevalent among Americans.

WHY WE AGE

Although researchers have a good understanding of how aging occurs, the forces that drive the aging process are a topic of some debate. Theories of aging fall into two general categories.

Programmed theories of aging say that, just like the factors that drive growth and maturation early in life, aging is a built-in process. It might be due to some predetermined switching on and off of certain genes that control biological processes. This biological clock may act through changes in hormone production, or through a decreasingly effective immune system or both. Proponents of this theory argue that aging *must* be programmed, as there isn't much variation in life span within a species.

One interesting bit of support for programmed aging dates back to the 1960s, when Dr. Leonard Hayflick from the Wistar Institute in Philadelphia experimented with cell reproduction in a laboratory culture. The cells of the body normally divide and reproduce in a process of constant renewal. At one time it was believed that cells themselves were immortal and could reproduce forever. Dr. Hayflick showed that this wasn't true. He found that certain cells eventually stop replicating and the cell line itself dies out.[2]

It was another three decades, however, before researchers discovered that a cell's life span appears to be determined by little tails of DNA that sit at the end of chromosomes. These DNA strands, called telomeres, shorten each time the cell divides. Once the telomeres are gone, the cell can no longer divide and it dies or becomes inactive.

Although telomere length is genetically determined, diet and lifestyle may have effects, too. In particular, oxidative stress (more on this in a minute) may lead to telomere shortening. And some preliminary research suggests that a program of comprehensive lifestyle change that includes exercise, stress management, and a near-vegan diet can have a positive effect on certain factors that impact telomere length.[3]

Telomeres don't seem to provide a complete explanation for aging, though. Some cells of the body don't divide over the life span, so wouldn't be affected by telomere length. But these cells still age. Clearly there are still many questions about the theory of programmed aging.

In contrast to this predetermined process of aging, other theories of aging put the focus more on environmental damage that accumulates over time (researchers refer to these as "error theories"). Environmental damage includes lifestyle factors that are well within our control. For example, high levels of blood glucose (blood sugar) can promote a process called glycation that results in protein molecules' bonding together and "cross-linking." Cross-linked proteins accumulate in tissues, where they reduce elasticity and affect overall function, and they are also responsible for some of the damage seen in aging skin and muscles and might also affect brain function.

Damage also occurs from production of unstable oxygen molecules called free radicals. These molecules are the result of normal metabolism—we are always generating free radicals—that can damage cells and interfere with their function. External factors, like UV radiation from sunlight and toxins from smoking, can also cause free radical production and oxidative damage. Oxidative damage might raise risk for many chronic diseases, such as heart disease, cancer, and Alzheimer's disease. It also promotes aging. Your body has antioxidant systems in place to neutralize free radicals, but if these systems become overwhelmed, the result is oxidative stress.

We know how to reduce oxidative damage and glycation, so it's likely that we can prevent premature aging through diet and lifestyle choices, slowing some age-related damage. For example, consuming foods that result in a more gradual and gentler elevation in blood glucose may reduce glycation and cross linking. We can also counter oxidative damage by flooding the body with compounds that neutralize free radicals and put a stop to oxidation. These compounds are antioxidants, and plant foods are rich sources of them. We'll talk more in the chapters ahead about food choices that can help to prevent glycation and oxidative damage.

AGING IS DIFFERENT FOR MEN AND WOMEN

Some of the changes seen in the fifty-plus body are related to declining levels in reproductive hormones—testosterone in men and estrogen in women. Because of the ways these hormone levels change, men and women may have different aging-related experiences.

TESTOSTERONE AND AGING IN MEN

Produced primarily in the testes, testosterone helps maintain bone density, fat distribution, muscle strength and mass, red blood cell production, and sperm production. In men, testosterone production declines gradually beginning at about age thirty, and then drops by about 1 percent per year.

The changes in sexual function, muscle strength, or mood that sometimes accompany changing hormone levels are likely to occur as subtle differences that aren't very obvious since the decline in testosterone is so gradual. Over time, though, lower levels of testosterone can contribute to poor bone health, depression, increased body fat and lower muscle mass, and changes in sexual function. In addition, testosterone deficiency is associated with type 2 diabetes, heart disease, stroke, and transient ischemic attacks (mini strokes).

But is the decline in testosterone levels truly inevitable? According to research on men in Australia, it isn't. In the Healthy Man Study, researchers looked at testosterone levels in 325 men between the ages of forty and ninety-seven. They found no changes in testosterone levels in men who said they were in good health, at least until their seventies.[4] It may be that lower testosterone levels are actually the consequence of chronic diseases, such as heart disease, and also of obesity, rather than the cause. If that's true, men may be able to put the brakes on declining testosterone levels with a healthy diet.

MENOPAUSE IN WOMEN

In contrast to what happens in men, it can feel as if estrogen levels in women fall with a thud as menopause approaches. While the menopause experience differs among women, it's a transition that doesn't go unnoticed. And there is no question about whether or not estrogen levels actually decline as women age. They do. It happens because the ovaries eventually run out of eggs, which causes them to stop producing the female sex hormones progesterone and estrogen.

Low estrogen levels can result in bone and muscle loss, thinning hair, and dry skin (and also eye and vaginal dryness). Some women also experience facial hair growth and skin breakouts. This is because women also produce small amounts of the male hormone testosterone. This doesn't decline with age, so after menopause, women have a higher ratio of testosterone to estrogen in their body than they did when they were younger. It sounds dismal, but there really are ways to mitigate many of these effects without resorting to hormone therapy or plastic surgery. You can protect the health of your muscles, bones, and skin with good diet and exercise choices.

Soy Foods, Menopause, and Hot Flashes

Although all women will notice changes that occur with estrogen decline, the hot flashes that we think of as synonymous with menopause affect just a little bit more than half of menopausal women. And researchers really aren't sure why they occur and precisely how they relate to lower estrogen levels.

It's interesting that Japanese women seldom complain of hot flashes. Whether this reflects cultural attitudes or the actual physical experience of menopause is something we don't know. Since higher-fiber diets are associated with somewhat lower blood levels of estrogen prior to menopause, this might present a benefit for those who eat more fiber-rich, plant-based diets.[5] The lower estrogen levels may represent a more gradual transition through menopause, preventing hot flashes. This would be helpful to women who consume a traditional Japanese diet, and also to vegan women. But the most promising theory is that it's their soy intake that gives Japanese women a little bit of advantage.

Soybeans and foods made from them contain phytochemicals called isoflavones that are a type of plant estrogen. They aren't exactly like the hormone estrogen that is produced in humans, though, because they are selective in the way they act. In certain tissues, isoflavones have effects similar to those of estrogen and in others they act as antiestrogens, eliciting opposite effects of estrogen. They also have effects that have nothing to do with estrogen.

When it comes to hot flashes, though, isoflavone effects appear to be beneficial, just like estrogen. The research suggests that isoflavones work to reduce both the frequency and severity of hot flashes.[6] More than fifty studies in the past two decades have looked at this phenomenon. It takes around 50 to 60 milligrams a day of isoflavones to reduce hot flashes, which is the amount found in about two servings of traditional soy foods (one serving is ½ cup of tofu, tempeh, edamame, or 1 cup of soy milk). Also, while there are many types of isoflavones in plants, the ones that are most prominent in soybeans and traditional soy foods such as tofu, tempeh, and soy milk appear to be the most effective in reducing hot flashes.[7] In contrast, veggie meats and other products made from soy protein tend to be low in isoflavones, which are usually lost in the process of making these foods.

Isoflavones may have other benefits for postmenopausal women, especially in regard to skin health—something we'll look at in chapter 5.

SOY FOODS FOR MEN

IF SOY ISOFLAVONES CAN help to counter some of the effects of declining estrogen in women, how do they affect men? Magazine articles and Internet posts have raised some concerns about this, suggesting their potential estrogen-like effects might cause feminine characteristics in men. Research doesn't bear this out, though.

An analysis of thirty-two clinical studies found that soy isoflavones had no significant effects on testosterone levels.[8] Studies also show that isoflavones don't adversely affect sperm or semen. For example, when healthy Western men took a daily supplement of 40 milligrams of isoflavones (about the amount that Japanese men typically consume), there was no effect on their hormone levels or semen concentration.[9] In fact, even when male subjects consumed as much as 480 milligrams of isoflavones per day—which is more than ten times the amount that the typical Japanese man consumes—there was no effect on sperm concentration.[10]

Popular news stories about men who experienced feminizing effects from eating soy foods have focused on just a couple of individuals who consumed enormous amounts of soy. In one case, nearly all of one young man's calories appeared to come from soy. The truth is that excessive intakes of any single food can lead to nutrient deficiencies and have negative effects on health. That's one reason why variety is an important rule in planning healthy diets.

Soy foods have been a mainstay of Asian diets for centuries with no apparent detrimental effects. They are often consumed beginning in infancy and then throughout life. Average intake differs among countries but is generally between one and two servings per day.[11] That can be a good guide for including soy foods in your own healthy diet.

HOW WE AGE

Aging is a universal process, and a relatively predictable one in humans. But it's also fairly variable among individuals. Yes, it's going to happen, but the rate of change is related in large part to factors that are under your control. Diet plays a big role and so do other lifestyle factors, such as exercise, sun protection, and stress management.

Let's look first at the kinds of changes that typically take place as people grow older, as understanding what happens and why makes it fairly easy to see how a healthy diet can affect these processes.

SKIN CHANGES

Your skin—which weighs in as the body's largest organ at about 6 pounds—shields your body from trauma, ultraviolet radiation, temperature extremes, toxins, and bacteria. It prevents entry of foreign substances and controls fluid losses. Skin is multilayered, containing blood vessels, hair follicles in some parts, sweat glands and nerves, fat cells, and proteins, such as collagen and elastin. Like every other part of your body, healthy skin needs good nutrition, especially plenty of vitamin A, vitamin C, zinc, and essential fats.

Because skin is constantly exposed to environmental damage and is also impacted by changes in hormones—and because it's simply more visible than other parts of the body—it's usually where we become most aware of the aging process. Skin becomes thinner with age, which is largely the consequence of slower cell regeneration. It takes as long as two months for skin cells to rejuvenate in older people compared to about one month in young adults.[12] Decreased synthesis of collagen results in loss of elasticity in the skin and more wrinkles. Older skin has fewer oil-producing glands and fewer blood vessels. In women there are fewer hormone receptors in the skin. These factors all affect how skin appears over the years. So does gravity.

Probably the single most damaging factor for skin health is sun exposure. It promotes oxidation and skin aging. Smoking also damages skin, and alcohol takes a toll in part because of its dehydrating effects.

COGNITIVE CHANGES

Your brain undergoes some changes with time, too, and these are perfectly normal—albeit annoying—consequences of aging. Neurological maturation peaks in the mid-20s, and then starts to decline gradually for several decades, and a little more quickly beginning in your sixties.

The changes that occur in the brain over time aren't fully understood but seem to involve a reduction in the size of neurons and in the number of neural synapses.[13] Synapses are connections between neurons through which information flows from one neuron to another.

Normal aging affects some aspects of brain function much more than others. For example, the memories that have been stored in your brain for many years will stick with you, whereas the ability to form new memories becomes impaired. That's why you can remember the name of the kid who sat next to you in kindergarten with ease, but maybe not the name of someone you met yesterday.

You might also find yourself feeling a bit less articulate than you used to be—not always able to find the word you need in conversation. The word is still there in your memory; it's the retrieval that takes a little more effort.

Interestingly, aging may actually enhance some brain functions. "Crystallized intelligence" involves accumulated knowledge and experience and long-term memory. This increases during your lifespan, assuming that you continue to learn and are exposed to new intellectual and cultural experiences. And there are things you can do to keep your brain sharp. Evidence suggests that you can continue to build new synapses by exercising your brain. (See 5 Ways to Exercise Your Brain on the next page.)

What most of us worry about, though, is overt dementia. Dementia is not a consequence of healthy aging; it's a disease—or, rather, a group of diseases. We'll talk more about it in chapter 6, when we look at dietary choices to prevent and manage chronic disease.

5 WAYS TO EXERCISE YOUR BRAIN

1. **Learn something new and challenging.** Try a new language or a musical instrument or a hobby, such as knitting, painting, dancing, or carpentry

2. **Play games that force your brain to work.** Sudoku, crossword puzzles, or Scrabble are all available on smart phones or tablets or your computer.

3. **Brush your teeth or write with your nondominant hand.** It gives your brain a workout!

4. **Get creative with words.** Write sonnets or haikus, or keep a journal, or write your autobiography for the grandkids.

5. **Put away your keyboard and grab a pen.** The act of writing may stimulate parts of the brain that enhance learning.

BODY COMPOSITION

Even if your weight doesn't change over the decades, you might feel as if things have shifted around a little bit. Hormone changes favor greater fat deposits and reduced muscle mass. Fat tissue also tends to accumulate in pockets, whereas it's more diffuse in younger people. It also migrates away from just beneath the skin to form deposits around the inner organs (visceral fat). As muscles age, they begin to shrink and the number and size of muscle fibers also decrease. Muscles become stiffer. Metabolism also slows with age, making it easier to put on weight.

The loss of muscle tissue that occurs with aging is an especially important public health problem. It can affect walking speed, balance, and, of course, strength. Poor muscle strength increases the risk of falling. Diets that are too low in protein and vitamin D can impact muscles and so can oxidative stress.

Bone metabolism changes as well. During the first four decades of life, bones are actively increasing in mass—and then for a decade or so, they stay about the same. Beginning in your midforties, bone losses start to outpace bone building and your skeleton becomes less dense and more fragile. Although men experience losses in bone mass as testosterone levels decline—and they can get osteoporosis, too— they start out with a higher bone density, giving them a little extra protection against fracture. Women are at greater risk for this disease as estrogen levels plummet at menopause. This combination of more fragile bones and poorer muscle strength raises risk for bone fracture. You can slow both muscle and bone loss, though, and even reverse loss once it has occurred as you'll see in chapter 5.

You may also find yourself losing an inch or two of height. This might be due to bone loss, but not necessarily. It can also be due to shrinking disks between the vertebrae. The cartilage that cushions joints between bones starts losing some of its water content, becoming susceptible to stress and degeneration, which can lead to arthritis.

EATING WELL: THE TASTE FACTOR

AGING DOESN'T JUST AFFECT our bones, muscles, hair, and skin. The number of taste buds on your tongue declines, too. In fact, taste sensation begins to dull a little bit beginning in early adulthood, but it happens more quickly after the age of seventy. As a result, food tastes blander and you might be tempted to add more and more sugar and salt to dishes over time. The answer is to seek out other assertive flavors:

▶ Boost the umami (see pages 49–50) in recipes with ingredients like sea veggies, sun-dried tomatoes, and dried mushrooms.

▶ Roasting or grilling foods also enhances umami, so try roasting vegetables instead of steaming them (see the Roasted Veggies recipe on page 280). Stock up on different types of vinegars. Balsamic vinegar has umami, and others, such as cider vinegar and especially seasoned rice vinegar, can perk up the flavors of any recipe. Try red wine or sherry vinegar in salad dressings and seasoned rice vinegar for stir-fried vegetables.

▶ Stir red wine into marinades and soups. Even just a few tablespoons enhances flavors beautifully.

▶ Flavor foods generously with whatever herbs and spices you especially enjoy. Don't be afraid to add more of an herb or spice than the recipe calls for. These plant-derived seasonings provide health promoting phytochemicals. They're good for you, so use as much as you need to make dishes flavorful and appealing.

▶ Flavor beans and roasted vegetables with liquid smoke for a burst of flavor.

▶ Use fruit to add sweetness to desserts so that your sugar comes from healthier foods. It's fine to use other sweeteners, too, but chopped fruit added to muffins and cakes can provide a little extra fiber and nutrition while satisfying your sweet tooth.

▶ Use sweeteners, such as maple syrup or molasses, that add their own unique flavors.

AGING IS PLASTIC:
A HEALTHY LIFESTYLE SLOWS THE HANDS OF TIME

The consequences of aging are normal and unavoidable. But it doesn't mean you can't continue to feel strong and energetic throughout your fifties and sixties and beyond. You can protect bone health, keep muscles strong, stay athletic if you choose, and avoid the worst offenders for aging skin. It's not some magical fountain of youth; rather, it is just a healthy lifestyle guided by good science.

Medical studies show that people can and do reverse some of the most common signs of aging, especially where bones and muscles are concerned. The prescription is not especially difficult either, and it won't have you buying all kinds of special supplements and face creams. Instead, it's a diet packed with plant proteins, fruits and veggies, and healthy fats, plus three inexpensive nutrient supplements. Add some good sunscreen, a little stress management, and lots of exercise for a lifestyle that will support health in the decades to come.

In the next chapter, we'll look at all of these elements of an anti-aging lifestyle and see how a healthy vegan diet can keep you energetic and vibrant.

VEGANS OVER 50 TELL THEIR STORIES

Athletic and Vegan | Greg Shaurette

Greg's story: Greg Shaurette and his wife are fifty-one and have been vegan since their early thirties. He became vegan in a rather circuitous route. Greg had always been athletic, and wanted to explore the impact of nutrition on his athletic endeavors.

As he began to learn about protein, fat, and carbohydrates, he reports, "It was clear to me that micronutrients, fiber, antioxidants, and phytochemicals were also important . . . I realized that if you want to get all of those other nutrients, you had to eat a wide variety of foods and mostly plants. Animal products simply took up too much space on the plate.

While gravitating toward a mostly plant-based plan, Greg says, "I came across the ethical arguments for veganism. They hit me like a ton of bricks. I'm the type of person who, once I know better, I am obligated to do better. It was when I was reading about dairy cows that I realized I was never going to consume animals again. I knew right then that I would never backslide. My then-girlfriend (now my wife) was totally into it as well. She is super compassionate and did not even need to hear all the right-brain reasons why eating animals was inappropriate.

"We have remained curious and have fine-tuned our diet over the years. We love to cook and eat a whole plant–based diet. The book *Becoming Vegan* was crucial during our early years, as was Ginny's book, *Vegan for Life*.

"We are a curiosity to some family members because they know how athletic we are and it bumps up against their understanding of nutrition. We feel the best thing we can do for the animals is be healthy and show others how doable veganism is. We frequently have houseguests and they know this is a vegan household. We serve them vegan meals, but they also know that if they need to go out to get a 'meat fix' that would be okay. We have never had anybody do that. In fact, they usually leave with an enlightened perspective about veganism. Many have made substantial changes in their own lives a result.

"At fifty-one we have peace of mind and healthy bodies. While many of our friends are acquiescing to 'getting old,' we don't feel any different than when we were in our twenties and thirties."

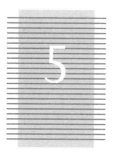

A HEALTHY DIET FOR 50+ VEGANS

NUTRIENT NEEDS CHANGE throughout the life span, and we need more of certain nutrients once we hit our fifties. Vegans and meat eaters alike will usually need supplements of vitamin B_{12} and vitamin D. Calcium requirements increase after age fifty, and so might needs for protein.

A few uncomplicated guidelines regarding food choices will help to ensure that you meet nutrient needs while also protecting the health of your brain, skin, muscles, and bones. It's a simple matter of choosing plenty of protein-rich plant foods, focusing on fruits and vegetables, choosing healthy fats, giving calcium intake a boost, and taking a few essential supplements.

> "My son and I are about to celebrate our one-year anniversary as vegans. It has been one of the best decisions we have ever made. It is all due to my son's persistence. He began talking to me at about age eleven or twelve about his desire to be vegetarian. After the third consecutive year, I told him he needed to bring me research demonstrating that he would get all the nutrients he needed. Fast forward . . . he educated me, we started out as vegetarians, and very quickly transitioned to veganism. He is fifteen and I just turned fifty-six!" —DIANNE

FRUITS AND VEGETABLES:
PACKED WITH NUTRIENTS AND ANTIOXIDANTS

Growing up, most of us knew that fruits and veggies provided nutrients like vitamin A for good eyesight, and vitamin C to ward off colds and the flu. Research from the past several decades has revealed that these foods have benefits that extend beyond their nutrient content, though. They are packed with plant chemicals—phytochemicals—that protect health and ward off chronic diseases, such as heart disease, hypertension, diabetes, and maybe cancer and Alzheimer's disease, too.

There are thousands of these plant chemicals in the foods we eat. Some may act together to protect against disease, too, so you can forget about trying to duplicate them in pills. All plant foods contain phytochemicals but fruits and vegetables are particularly rich sources.

Some phytochemicals are antioxidants—the compounds that counter oxidative damage to cells. They may slow aging in the skin, muscles, and brain. For example, compounds called anthocyanins, which are especially abundant in berries, are being studied for possible protection against dementia. Evidence for their protective role comes from the Nurse's Health Study, an ongoing study of the health of more than 200,000 female nurses.

The investigators began measuring cognitive function in 16,010 participants who had been filling out questionnaires about their food intake every two years, beginning in 1980. At the start of the study, there was little difference in cognitive function among the women. However, over time, those who consumed the most blueberries and strawberries and therefore had the highest intake of anthocyanins, showed slower declines in cognitive function in their seventies. Those with the highest intakes—they consumed blueberries at least once a week and strawberries at least twice per week—delayed cognitive aging by about two and a half years. The anthocyanins in these foods may accumulate in the parts of the brain that control learning and memory where they could provide protection through their antioxidant and anti-inflammatory properties.[1]

Antioxidants may also protect skin from sun damage. Beta-carotene, a compound that our body converts to vitamin A, is an antioxidant that is abundant in foods like carrots and leafy green vegetables. Lycopene is an antioxidant in tomatoes. Both of these compounds accumulate in skin and can reduce damaging effects of the sun's UV radiation.[2] Eating these foods isn't the equivalent of slathering on a good sunscreen, but evidence indicates that they add at least one layer of protection against sun damage.

Eating more veggies may help to keep eyesight sharp as you get older, too. Corn, spinach, kale, and broccoli are all especially rich in two powerful compounds: lutein and zeaxanthin. These pigments accumulate in the macula of the eye's retina. Lutein gives the macula its yellow hue (lutea is Latin for "yellow") and both compounds filter out harmful UV rays and are associated with decreased risk for macular degeneration. Macular degeneration is a chronic eye disease that causes vision loss in the center of the field of vision.

Overall, vegans may have fewer vision-related problems as they age, probably because of their higher intake of antioxidants. One large British study found that compared to regular meat eaters, lacto-ovo vegetarians were 30 percent less likely to have cataracts, and vegans had a 40 percent lower risk.[3]

In addition to phytochemicals, many of the nutrients in fruits and vegetables also play crucial roles in keeping your body healthy. Leafy green vegetables, like spinach, kale, and collards, are among the best dietary sources of vitamin K, which is needed for healthy bones. Higher intakes of vitamin K are associated with lower rates of hip fractures and greater bone density.[4] Vitamin C from citrus fruits and green vegetables also protects bone health. In fact, eating more fruits and vegetables is associated with better bone health at all stages of life—adolescence through the later years.[5] The minerals potassium and magnesium also promote bone strength, and vegans often have much higher intakes of both of these nutrients.

HEALTHY PLANT FOODS: THE BEST OF THE BEST

All whole plant foods are good for you. But you'll see that certain foods are mentioned over and over in this book, especially in relationship to planning healthy vegan diets and reducing risk for chronic disease. You don't *have* to eat each and every one of the following foods. Skip the ones that don't appeal to you. But for the ones you enjoy, include them in meals often. We made a point of featuring these foods in our recipes.

TABLE 2-1: HEALTHY PLANT FOODS: THE BEST OF THE BEST

	RICH IN PROTEIN FOR STRONG MUSCLES AND BONES	PROVIDE CALCIUM FOR HEALTHY BONES	HIGH IN POTASSIUM TO KEEP BLOOD PRESSURE LOW AND PROTECT BONE AND HEART HEALTH	PACKED WITH PHYTOCHEMICALS THAT REDUCE RISK FOR CANCER	GREAT SOURCE OF RESISTANT STARCH AND FIBER TO LOWER BLOOD CHOLESTEROL AND CONTROL DIABETES	SOURCE OF SLOW CARBS TO KEEP BLOOD GLUCOSE LEVELS HEALTHY	PROVIDE GOOD FATS FOR A HEALTHY HEART	PACKED WITH COMPOUNDS THAT PROTECT COGNITION
All types of dried beans, peas, and lentils	X		X		X			
Tofu, tempeh, edamame, soy milk	X	X	X	X				
Seitan (wheat meat)	X							
Sweet potatoes						X		
Quinoa	X					X		
Barley, oats, pasta					X	X		
Cooked tomato products				X (especially for prostate cancer)				

	RICH IN PROTEIN FOR STRONG MUSCLES AND BONES	PROVIDE CALCIUM FOR HEALTHY BONES	HIGH IN POTASSIUM TO KEEP BLOOD PRESSURE LOW AND PROTECT BONE AND HEART HEALTH	PACKED WITH PHYTOCHEMICALS THAT REDUCE RISK FOR CANCER	GREAT SOURCE OF RESISTANT STARCH AND FIBER TO LOWER BLOOD CHOLESTEROL AND CONTROL DIABETES	SOURCE OF SLOW CARBS TO KEEP BLOOD GLUCOSE LEVELS HEALTHY	PROVIDE GOOD FATS FOR A HEALTHY HEART	PACKED WITH COMPOUNDS THAT PROTECT COGNITION
Raw broccoli and cabbage				X				
Kale, collard greens, turnip greens, bok choy		X		X				
Spinach, corn, Swiss chard, beet greens			X (spinach and corn protect eye health, too)					
Berries								X
Figs		X						
Bananas					X			
Peanuts and peanut butter	X							X
Flaxseeds, walnuts, chia seeds, hemp seeds, canola oil							X (for essential omega-3 fats)	
Almonds and almond butter		X					X	
Extra virgin olive oil							X	
Fortified almond, coconut, and rice milk		X						

OMEGA-3 FATS FOR YOUR SKIN AND HEART

Two fatty acids in foods are essential nutrients, which means they are absolutely required in the diet. One, called linoleic (lin oh LAY ik) acid, is a member of the omega-6 family of fats. It's abundant in all kinds of plant foods; certain vegetable oils, such as corn and soy oil, are particularly rich in this fat. You really never have to worry about getting enough linoleic acid. A vegan diet will provide plenty of it without any effort from you.

The other essential fat is alpha-linolenic (lin oh LEN ik) acid (ALA), which is a member of the omega-3 family of fats. It's found in only a handful of plant foods, so while you don't need much of it, you do need to pay attention to food sources. Flaxseeds are an especially good source of this nutrient. They have a hard outer shell that resists digestion, so purchase ground flaxseeds or flaxseed meal or grind whole seeds in a coffee grinder. Be sure to store it in the freezer to protect it from going rancid.

You can sprinkle flaxseed meal on oatmeal or any type of grain or blend it into smoothies. It also makes a wonderful egg replacer in baking (see page 225). Chia and hemp are other tiny seeds that provide ALA. (Although hemp is part of the cannabis family, the plants grown for food don't have the druglike properties of marijuana.)

You can also get your daily dose of ALA by sprinkling a few teaspoons of chopped walnuts on cereal or by dressing a salad with a vinaigrette made with walnut oil. Soy foods also provide small amounts, and leafy green vegetables provide a little bit of this fat, too, although not enough to meet your ALA needs on their own.

Some vegan diets that are ultra-low in fat may fall short of needs for alpha-linolenic acid. It's important to make sure you're including at least one good food source of this fat in your diet every day. ALA is especially important for healthy skin and it may also help reduce risk for heart disease.

Table 2-2 shows how easy it is to meet ALA needs.

TABLE 2-2: FOODS TO MEET DAILY ALA NEEDS

	WOMEN	MEN
Walnut, soy, or canola oil	1 tablespoon	4 teaspoons
Flaxseed oil	¾ teaspoon	1 teaspoon
Hemp seed oil	2 teaspoons	3 teaspoons
Walnuts	3 walnut halves	4 walnut halves
Ground flaxseeds	3 teaspoons	4 teaspoons
Chia seeds	1½ teaspoons	2 teaspoons

The omega-3 family of fats also includes DHA (docosahexaenoic acid) and EPA (eicosapentaenoic acid). You've probably heard about these fats because they are the ones that are abundant in fatty fish and fish oil supplements. They aren't considered essential because humans can synthesize them from the essential fat ALA—the one found in flaxseeds, hemp seeds, and walnuts. So technically, if you are eating enough ALA, you'll make enough DHA and EPA. The reality, though, is that production of DHA and EPA is not very efficient, especially as we age.

People who don't have direct sources of these fats in their diets, including vegans, have lower blood levels of DHA and EPA.[6] But does it matter? That's something nutrition experts don't know. There is evidence that DHA and EPA help to protect cognitive function with aging and also may reduce risk for heart disease.[7] They may also be valuable in reducing depression and in helping to reduce symptoms of painful conditions, such as rheumatoid arthritis.[8] However, that evidence is conflicting and these are topics of ongoing research with no real consensus among the experts.

For now, with the issue unresolved, it may make sense to take a small daily supplement of these fats. Fortunately, you don't need to eat fish or take fishy-tasting supplements to get them. Fish get their DHA and EPA by eating microalgae, and we can get them from the same source. Supplements providing algae-derived DHA and EPA are a much better option for getting these fats for anyone, vegan or not, since they are a better choice for the environment. Ginny recommends a daily supplement that provides between 200 and 300 milligrams of DHA and EPA combined.

GOOD NUTRITION FROM NUTS AND SEEDS

Although there are only a few nuts and seeds that provide essential omega-3 fats, other choices from this food group—cashews, pistachios, almonds, hazelnuts, Brazil nuts, pecans, sunflower seeds, and pumpkin seeds—have their own benefits. Many are good sources of minerals such as zinc, a nutrient that helps to protect skin and the immune system. Almonds and pistachios are both rich in protein, and almonds also provide calcium.

Since seeds are the source of all plant life, it's not surprising that they, too, offer an abundance of nutrients. Certain ones, such as sunflower seeds, are especially rich in vitamin E, an important antioxidant nutrient.

Nuts and seeds are both also good sources of healthy fats, and you'll see in chapter 6 that nuts in particular play important roles in chronic disease prevention. Add them to salads for a little extra flavor, crunch, and nutrition. And don't overlook the butters made from nuts and seeds. Almond butter is a favorite on toast or spread on celery sticks or apple slices. Tahini, which is sesame seed butter, is an essential ingredient in hummus. Thinned with fresh lemon juice and water, it also makes a delicious dressing for leafy green salads or a sauce for vegetables or grains. (See page 249 for our Basic Hummus recipe.)

A serving of these foods is ¼ cup of whole nuts or 2 tablespoons of seeds, chopped nuts, or nut or seed butter. Depending on your calorie needs, aim for one to two servings of these foods per day.

VITAMIN B$_{12}$: NOT JUST FOR VEGANS

Vitamin B$_{12}$ is the big nutrition issue in vegan diets. Because it's found only in animal foods, vegans need to take supplements or use fortified foods. But, for people over the age of fifty, vitamin B$_{12}$ is not just a vegan issue, because even those who eat meat need supplements.

In animal foods, vitamin B$_{12}$ is bound to protein. When B$_{12}$ arrives in the stomach, it's released from its protein carrier, a necessary step before it can be absorbed into the blood. Changes in stomach secretions that occur with aging, however, make it increasingly difficult to break the bond between B$_{12}$ and its protein carrier. As a result, many people over the age of fifty may not absorb vitamin B$_{12}$ very well.

Since vitamin B$_{12}$ is crucial for a healthy nervous system, even subtle deficiencies can impact hearing, balance, and memory. And the B$_{12}$ deficiency may go unnoticed if people think that what they are experiencing are just normal signs of aging. Low vitamin B$_{12}$ is also linked to poorer bone health and to increased risk for heart disease.[9]

The solution is a simple one—a B$_{12}$ supplement. The type of vitamin B$_{12}$ found in supplements and fortified foods is not bound to protein and is absorbed much more easily than the vitamin B$_{12}$ found in animal foods. Vegans always need to take vitamin B$_{12}$ supplements or use fortified foods because plant foods don't provide this vitamin. But so do meat-eaters over the age of fifty, as many may not be able to absorb the protein-bound B$_{12}$ in animal foods.

Make sure you get enough vitamin B$_{12}$ by taking a supplement or by eating two or three servings per day of a food that is fortified with vitamin B$_{12}$. Despite claims to the contrary in some popular books and on the Internet, you can't get vitamin B$_{12}$ by eating unwashed organic vegetables or by eating sea vegetables or algae, such as spirulina. Fermented soy foods won't provide B$_{12}$, either.

Look for supplements that are in the form of cyanocobalamin, which is the type that has been studied the most. Many supplements contain methylcobalamin, which may not be quite as stable as the cyano form, so it's not as reliable for protecting your B_{12} levels. Take a daily supplement providing between 25 and 100 micrograms or take a pill providing 1,000 micrograms three times per week. Look for tablets that are chewable (most are) to maximize absorption. As with other supplements, when shopping for them, look for "suitable for vegetarians" or "vegan" on the label, as some supplements may contain small amounts of animal ingredients as fillers.

Many veggie meats and plant-based milks are fortified with vitamin B_{12}. If you rely on fortified foods for this nutrient, aim for two servings per day of foods that provide at least 1.5 micrograms of B_{12}. Eat these foods several hours apart to ensure adequate absorption of this vitamin.

PLANT PROTEINS FOR MUSCLES AND BONES

It is estimated that about 40 percent of American men and women over the age of fifty fall short of the recommended dietary allowance (RDA) of protein, despite the fact that most eat meat.[10] It's probable that this shortfall is one of the reasons that declining muscle mass is so common among older Americans. The two most important factors for slowing that loss are adequate protein and plenty of exercise.[11]

Because protein may be used less efficiently with aging, the current recommendations for adults might not protect muscle mass in older people.[12] In one study of two thousand men and women, those who had protein intakes that were about a third higher than the RDA lost far less muscle after the age of seventy compared to people whose protein intake was just shy of the RDA.[13]

Protein is also important for bone health. A couple of decades ago, we thought that just the opposite was true—that higher protein intake was harmful to bone health. It's a belief that was based on a 1992 study that compared hip fracture rates around the world. The study showed that people were least likely to break a hip if they lived in a country where animal protein was typically low. One theory was that higher protein intake created a more acidic environment in the body that drew calcium out of bones.

We know now that this isn't true. The low rates of hip fracture in certain countries seem to have more to do with culture and ethnicity than diet. For example, better balance and strength among some of these populations means that people are less likely to fall and therefore less likely to break a bone. And there are also differences in hip anatomy among different ethnic groups that give certain groups a little bit of protection against fractures regardless of their diet. In fact, in some countries where hip fracture rates are low, people actually have more osteoporosis, especially in their spine.

The evidence now points to a protective effect of protein on bones.[14] Protein enhances calcium absorption from the diet—which is good for bones—and is also an important part of the bone structure. Protein also promotes strong muscles, which in turn keep bones strong.

The Adventist Health Study, a large-scale study of American vegetarians, looked at the relationship of protein intake to the risk for fractures in nearly two thousand women. The researchers looked specifically at wrist fractures and found that vegetarian women who ate the most protein-rich foods, such as beans, soy foods, and veggie meats, were 68 percent less likely to experience a wrist fracture.[15] In the Iowa Women's Health Study, which followed the health of more than forty thousand postmenopausal women, higher protein intake was associated with lower rates of hip fracture.[16]

The key to packing your vegan diet with protein is to eat at least four servings of legumes per day. If that sounds like a lot, keep in mind that legumes are much more than just beans. This group of foods includes the huge array of soy foods, such as tofu, edamame, tempeh, soy milk, and veggie meats. Legumes also include peanuts and peanut butter. And a serving size is small—just ½ cup of cooked beans or tofu, or ¼ cup of peanuts or 2 tablespoons of peanut butter.

Getting protein from plants is smart because it comes packaged with fiber and phytochemicals; you won't find either in meat. Plant proteins may also help to protect kidney function, which can decline with age.[17] And you'll see in chapter 6 that soy foods may have benefits in reducing chronic disease risk. This may help to explain the lower rates of some chronic diseases in countries such as Japan and China.

---

5 THINGS TO DO WITH CANNED BEANS

OPEN UP A CAN of beans, and dinner is almost ready. Here are five super quick things you can do with canned beans.

1. Mix taco seasoning into canned black beans. Spread them on a corn tortilla and heat in the oven or microwave. Top with chopped tomatoes, cubes of avocado, and spicy salsa.
2. Stir frozen corn and chopped onion into pinto beans. Serve on a bed of quinoa or brown rice.
3. Mix Sloppy Joe sauce into cannellini beans, then heat and serve over whole wheat vegan hamburger buns.
4. Gently mash drained, canned chickpeas and add vegan mayonnaise and chopped onion and celery. Serve in a sandwich or on top of a bed of fresh greens.
5. Sauté chopped onions in extra virgin olive oil. Add a can of black-eyed peas and a pinch of cayenne pepper.

FRIENDLY BACTERIA FROM BEANS

If beans give you gas, it's actually very easy to avoid this problem. The gas comes from small sugars or carbohydrates called oligosaccharides that are abundant in beans. You can reduce oligosaccharides by giving the beans a long overnight soak in lots of water in the refrigerator. Pour off the water the next day; you'll be pouring off most of the oligosaccharides—as much as three-quarters of the total.[18] Adding a pinch of baking soda to the cooking water reduces the oligosaccharide content even further.

If you're not bothered by gas from eating beans, though, consider cooking them without the presoak. Those oligosaccharides are actually good for you. They promote the growth of healthy bacteria in the colon, which may reduce risk for colon cancer.[19] According to *World Vegan Feast* author Bryanna Clark Grogan, who has studied the soaking issue extensively, a few types of beans—favas, soybeans, and chick-peas—will usually benefit from an overnight soak, as they take too long to cook otherwise. Other kinds of beans—black, kidney, pinto, and navy beans, for example—can be cooked without soaking.

CALCIUM-RICH FOODS FOR BONE HEALTH

The idea of getting calcium without milk seems a little foreign to those of us who grew up—and in some cases spent many of our adult years—depending on cow's milk, yogurt, and cheese for this mineral. But milk drinking is a relatively new human habit, and it's actually very uncommon in some parts of the world. In fact, normal human development makes it difficult to drink milk for many people. Humans require an enzyme called lactase to digest the sugar in milk, and it's normal and common for the body to stop producing this enzyme after childhood. Nature makes sure we are pumping out plenty of lactase in infancy because we need it to digest breast milk. After that, levels start to decline. It doesn't mean we no longer need calcium. It suggests however that we are supposed to be looking toward other foods to get it.

For our ancestors, those other foods were wild greens. Many of the greens that they foraged for are no longer available—although some of the weeds you pluck out of your garden are descendants of those early wild plants. But there are excellent choices at your grocery store, such as kale, collards, and turnip and mustard greens. Some soy foods are also good sources of calcium.

In the United States, most plant-based milks—those made from soy, almonds, and hemp seeds—are fortified with calcium, providing about the same amount per cup that you'd get from cow's milk. And of course, fortified orange juice is an easy way to increase your calcium intake.

Although not the healthiest foods in the world, in a pinch—especially when you're on the go—a vegan protein bar, such as a Luna Bar, will give you a fast dose of calcium and protein. Other foods that provide calcium include navel oranges, almond butter, tahini, white beans, and figs. Blackstrap molasses can also provide calcium to your diet—about 80 milligrams in a tablespoon. Don't confuse it with regular molasses, which doesn't provide calcium. Blackstrap molasses is more concentrated and has a very robust flavor. Small amounts can be used to sweeten hot cereal or for baking. Some vegetables like broccoli and cabbage will contribute small amounts of calcium to your diet, too.

OUR VEGAN LIVES

How We Heed Nutritional Advice: Eat Your Greens

Patti: I like to include as many excellent choices as I can early in the day. So I usually make a green smoothie in the morning (see page 241) and nurse it until lunchtime. And for breakfast I often have oatmeal with berries or other fruit and ground flaxseeds and walnuts. Because my morning time in the kitchen is so routine, this breakfast and beverage take less than 5 minutes to prepare. And if I know that I'll be rushed in the morning, I prepare it all the night before and simply heat the oatmeal and blend the smoothie as soon as I wake up.

To maximize my intake of greens, I will add chopped kale or collards to most of the soups I make and add more greens each time I reheat the soup. And I've learned that just about any salad can be made more nutrient dense with the addition of a few chopped leaves of spinach, kale, or collards. Also on sandwiches, I use kale or collards in place of lettuce—except on vegan BLTs.

Carol: For many years, I knew the refrain "All greens are good for you," yet I didn't set myself any goals for adding more greens to my diet. I really began to take eating greens more seriously as Patti and I worked on our earlier book, How to Eat Like a Vegetarian. So, I started the discipline of bringing home chard, kale, or collard greens and trying to prepare them in ways that Patti and I were discussing. Patti likes to put some peanut butter on collard greens and roll them up, so I tried that. A breakthrough for me came when I tried a massaged kale salad (see page 260); it was delicious and easy. Another way I discovered for preparing kale was to remove its stems, tear it into bite-size pieces, toss with a tablespoon or two of oil, and roast for 6 to 7 minutes in a 375°F oven. Even non-kale lovers seem won over by that.

Ginny: Frozen spinach was the only leafy green veggie I ever saw when I was growing up. I never even heard of kale, collards, chard, or turnip greens. Today, these foods are a major part of my diet. I depend on kale and collards for the calcium they provide and I eat them almost every day. And I like to pack lots of spinach into dishes for some extra protein and potassium.

I eat both fresh and frozen greens and I eat the fresh ones raw and cooked. There is always a bag of frozen chopped spinach in the freezer so that I can add it to lentil soup or stir it into cooked quinoa. My lunch is a big salad every day and I tuck all kinds of raw greens into that, including baby spinach and baby kale.

When I have greens for dinner I'll often top them with a spicy homemade sauce or one from a bottle, or stir-fry them quickly in a little olive oil with a pinch of cayenne and garlic.

CALCIUM FROM PLANTS

The calcium RDA for people over the age of fifty is 1,200 milligrams per day. It may be quite a bit more than some people need, as nutrient needs vary among individuals. But when it comes to protecting your bone health, you might as well err on the side of caution. In fact, higher amounts of calcium can be effective in reducing bone loss or preventing fractures in people over the age of fifty.[20]

US government guidelines recommend two to three servings of dairy foods per day as a way to meet calcium needs. That's one way to get calcium, and you could do pretty much the same by drinking two to three glasses of fortified almond or soy milk. But, variety is, after all, a cornerstone of healthy and pleasurable eating, so why not get your calcium from small servings of lots of different foods. Any of the following foods would provide about 150 milligrams of calcium:

- ½ cup of fortified soy, almond, or hemp seed milk
- ½ cup of calcium-fortified orange juice
- ½ cup of tofu made with calcium sulfate
- ½ cup of calcium-fortified soy, almond, or coconut yogurt
- 1 cup of cooked bok choy, collards, kale, mustard greens, or turnip greens
- ½ cup of Chinese cabbage or mustard greens
- 1 cup of white beans
- 2 tablespoons of almond butter or sesame tahini
- ¼ cup of almonds
- 2 navel oranges
- ½ cup of dried figs

Many other foods provide small amounts of calcium, too. So, if you mix and match the foods in this list to provide around 1,000 milligrams of calcium, you'll have no trouble ending up with the 1,200 milligrams recommended for people over the age of fifty. If you find that you routinely fall short of meeting calcium needs, it's fine to make up the difference with a low-dose calcium supplement. Aim to get as much of your calcium as possible from foods, though. Here are two examples of daily menus that provide about 1,200 milligrams of calcium.

MENU 1

- ▶ BREAKFAST: 1 cup of oatmeal with ½ cup of fortified soy milk
- ▶ SNACK: bagel spread with 2 tablespoons of almond butter
- ▶ LUNCH: vegan bean soup made with 1 cup of white beans
- ▶ DINNER: tofu stir-fry with ½ cup of tofu and 1½ cups of bok choy

MENU 2

- ▶ BREAKFAST: smoothie (1 cup of fortified almond milk, 2 tablespoons of peanut butter, ½ frozen banana, and pinches of ground nutmeg and cinnamon)
- ▶ SNACK: 1 cup of soy yogurt with fresh strawberries
- ▶ LUNCH: vegan lentil soup, 1 cup of calcium-fortified orange juice
- ▶ DINNER: bean burrito with a tossed salad

LEARNING TO LOVE GREENS

DEPENDING ON WHERE YOU grew up, you may or may not know leafy green vegetables very well. You don't absolutely have to eat them to be healthy, but greens are incredibly nutritious. And once you know what to do with them, you'll find that being introduced to leafy greens is one of those nice little health and culinary perks that comes with a new vegan lifestyle.

Leafy greens can be divided roughly into two categories, with somewhat different nutritional strengths. The cruciferous veggies—members of the cabbage family—include collards, kale, turnip greens, bok choy, and mustard greens. They're loaded with calcium, which is one reason why these foods—especially kale and collards—play such a big role in many vegan diets.

Spinach, chard, and beet greens are members of the chenopod family. These are more delicate greens that cook up quickly. They contain calcium, too, but it's bound to compounds called oxalates that prevent the calcium from being absorbed. What the chenopods do provide in abundance is potassium, a mineral that is important for bone strength and that helps to protect against heart disease. Spinach, chard, and beet greens have much more potassium than do cruciferous greens.

All of these leafy greens are good sources of vitamin A and also vitamin K. And some from each group—collards, turnip greens, and spinach—are rich in the B vitamin folate. Kale and spinach both provide lutein, the phytochemical that protects eyesight.

Bottom line: All greens are good for you, so if you like them, eat them often and eat a variety.

VITAMIN D PROTECTS MUSCLES, BONES, AND BRAIN FUNCTION

Vitamin D is an oddity in the world of nutrition. It's really not a nutrient at all. It's basically a hormone, and—technically—we have no requirement for it in the diet. That's because we can make what we need when skin is exposed to sunlight. It's obvious that we evolved to get our vitamin D this way because there is hardly any of it in foods. A few types of fish are natural sources of vitamin D but it's neither practical nor sustainable to get vitamin D this way. You may have thought that cow's milk is a good source of vitamin D but that is only because it's fortified with it. So everyone—no matter his or her diet—is getting vitamin D exactly the same way—from supplements, fortified foods, or sunlight.

Vitamin D protects bone health by enhancing calcium absorption and reducing calcium losses in the urine. Vitamin D is also important for muscle strength, which in turn can improve bone health. Strong muscles also make it less likely that you will fall and fracture a bone. In older people, adding vitamin D to the diet can reduce risk of falling by as much as 20 percent.[21] But vitamin D seems to have effects that

reach far beyond bones and muscle strength. It may have roles in reducing risk for heart disease,[22] diabetes,[23] colon cancer,[24] multiple
sclerosis,[25] dementia,[26] and depression.[27] It's also important for the
immune system and for skin health.

SUPPLEMENTS VERSUS SUNLIGHT FOR VITAMIN D

The amount of vitamin D you make from exposure to sunlight depends
on many factors—your skin tone, where you live (even in warmer climates smog and clouds interfere with vitamin D synthesis), and how
much of your skin is exposed to the sun. Not surprisingly, many older
people have vitamin D levels that are too low since the ability to synthesize vitamin D decreases with aging.[28] Young adults may make as much
as four times the amount of vitamin D compared to older adults.[29]

People with darker skin also make vitamin D less easily. It can take
as much as six times the amount of sun exposure to raise blood levels
of vitamin D in dark-skinned people compared to those with a fairer
skin tone.[30] And whatever your age or skin tone, it's next to impossible
to make enough vitamin D during the winter months if you live far
from the equator.

Because vitamin D synthesis decreases with age, you may need increasingly greater exposure to sunlight to make enough. And you'll
need to weigh the benefits of that exposure against the risks. Exposure
to sunlight causes photoaging, which is sun-induced skin aging. And
while lighter-skinned individuals need less sun exposure to make vitamin D, they are also more prone to sun-induced skin damage.

This damage doesn't just affect your appearance, of course. It also
greatly raises your risk for skin cancer. UV radiation from sunlight is
a significant carcinogen. And because chances are that you won't end
up making enough vitamin D anyway—even people living in sunny
climates often have levels of vitamin D that are too low[31]—it makes far
more sense to slather on some sunscreen to protect your skin and take
a supplement to protect your vitamin D status.

The RDA for vitamin D is 600 IUs (international units) for adults up to the age of seventy and then it rises to 800 IUs per day. Some health experts believe that somewhat higher intakes are beneficial, although that's controversial. Supplements usually provide between 1,000 and 2,000 IUs per dose, and you can safely take that amount.

Vitamin D2 Versus Vitamin D3

Most supplements contain vitamin D_3, also called cholecalciferol, which is almost always derived from either lanolin—a product of sheep's wool—or fish oil. Vitamin D_2 or ergocalciferol, is a vegan version of vitamin D derived from yeast. It's increasingly available as a supplement and is also used to fortify many plant-based milks. Either form will protect your vitamin D status.

Some research suggests however, that vitamin D_2 stays in your blood for a shorter period of time—just a few days as opposed to a few weeks for vitamin D_3. When people are treated for vitamin D deficiency, they are sometimes given megadoses of the vitamin every week or so. In that case, vitamin D_3 might be more effective for treatment. If you're taking a daily supplement of vitamin D, however, then vitamin D_2 is just as beneficial.[32] Recently, vitamin D_3 has been produced from lichen—a vegan source of this form of the vitamin.

WHOLE GRAINS DELIVER FIBER AND MINERALS

Humans have been eating grains for at least ten thousand years—corn in Central America, rice in Asia, quinoa in the Andes, and wheat in Africa and the Middle East. Even before the advent of agriculture, hunter-gatherers may have included small amounts of grains in their diet. But they ate only whole grains, of course. Industrialized roller mills, which strip away the bran and germ from grains, weren't in use until around 150 years ago.

Milled grains have long been valued because they don't get rancid and they produce light and airy baked products. Unfortunately, milling also strips away vitamins, minerals, and fiber. It makes grains more digestible, too, which is not a good thing. More easily digested refined grains cause blood glucose levels to rise too rapidly. Over time, this may raise risk for some chronic diseases, including type 2 diabetes. Whole grains are important sources of minerals, such as zinc and iron, in vegan diets. Both are absorbed at a lower rate from grains because these foods are also rich in phytates, compounds that bind to minerals and reduce their absorption. Phytates aren't all bad; they are antioxidants and may have some health benefits. And you can counter their effects on nutrient absorption with a few simple preparation methods. Sprouting grains increases mineral absorption, and so does leavening whole-grain flour with yeast or a vegan sourdough starter to make bread. For iron, consuming grains along with vitamin C–rich foods will boost absorption.

Whole grains also provide vitamin B_6, a nutrient we need in higher amounts after age fifty. Most vegans get plenty of this nutrient, but including a few servings of whole grains in your diet every day is a good way to ensure adequate vitamin B_6 intake.

It's okay to have occasional refined grains, but choose whole grains most of the time. In chapter 6 we'll talk a little bit more about how to make the best whole-grain choices to keep blood glucose levels healthy.

CALORIE NEEDS AND WEIGHT MANAGEMENT

Meeting nutrient needs on a vegan diet is easy once you know the basics. But for those of us over fifty, regardless of the type of diet we eat, there is a little bit of a challenge to balancing calorie needs against nutritional needs. While our requirements for some nutrients increase over time, our calorie needs may decline. It means we need to pack a lot of nutrition into fewer calories.

A drop in calorie needs may be the consequence of a slower metabolism that comes with normal aging. But part of the explanation is also a decrease in muscle mass along with the fact that some people slack off on physical activity over time. The answer is obviously to be more physically active. Weight training helps build muscle mass, and aerobic exercise, such as walking, jogging, bicycling, or Zumba, burns lots of calories. You don't have to be an athlete, but the more you get up and move around, the more calories you can consume without gaining weight, which makes it easier to meet your nutritional needs.

Vegans may have a little bit of an edge in preventing the pounds from piling on. Our higher-fiber diet slows digestion and may help to prevent hunger.[33] Plant eaters also have different types of bacteria living in their colon. Everyone harbors colonies of microorganisms in their lower intestine, but the type of bacteria varies depending on diet. There is some evidence that the type of bacteria in vegetarian colons is associated with improved weight management.[34]

Phytochemicals in fruits and vegetables are also associated with better weight management by increasing activity of enzymes that induce fat breakdown and that promote energy expenditure.[35]

WHERE TO LEARN MORE ABOUT NUTRITION

THIS CHAPTER PROVIDES YOU with the basic information you need to stay healthy on your vegan diet. If you want a little more in-depth information, here are some of Ginny's highly recommended resources for accurate vegan nutrition information:

WEBSITES

TheVeganRD.com (this is Ginny's blog)
veganhealth.org
vegetariannutrition.net
jacknorrisrd.com
vrg.org

BOOKS

Vegan for Her by Virginia Messina with JL Fields
Vegan for Life by Jack Norris and Virginia Messina
Simply Vegan, 5th edition, by Debra Wasserman and Reed Mangels
Becoming Vegan by Brenda Davis and Vesanto Melina

The Plant-Powered Diet by Sharon Palmer
Defeating Diabetes by Brenda Davis and Tom Barnard

HEALTHY HABITS AT ANY SIZE

While there are factors that give vegans some small advantages, a vegan diet is not a guaranteed slenderizing plan. If you find your weight creeping up with age, you may find that a combination of going vegan and giving your exercise a little boost is enough to put the brakes on weight gain. If you've struggled with weight all of your life, then things are a little bit more complicated.

Truthfully, the one and only guaranteed plan for permanent weight loss—an approach that works for everyone—isn't known. There are so many factors that affect weight, including genetics and environmental impacts. So, you may have jumped around from one diet to another, losing and then regaining weight. That's not especially good for you physically or psychologically.

A better approach is to toss out the scale and switch your focus away from weight toward optimal health. Engaging in regular exercise and choosing healthy foods can improve your health at any body size. For example, in the Dietary Alternatives to Stop Hypertension (DASH) Study, people who ate more fruits and vegetables and less saturated fat experienced reductions in blood pressure even when they didn't lose weight.[36]

Other research shows that a healthy lifestyle that produces small weight loss—about 5 percent of body weight—translates to significant improvements in health. At the Pritikin Longevity Center, people who ate a low-fat, high-fiber diet and who exercised regularly experienced improvements in blood pressure, cholesterol levels, and blood glucose control that were far greater that what could be explained by their small weight loss.[37]

What these and other studies show us is that, as much as we might desire to be thin, it's being healthy that really matters. Your "healthy body weight" is the weight that you can realistically maintain and at which you enjoy good health.

And research doesn't support the idea that you need to be skinny to be healthy. While obesity is associated with higher risk for some diseases, being a little bit overweight isn't. When a group of US and Canadian researchers analyzed data from ninety-seven studies that included close to 3 million people, they found that carrying a few extra pounds was associated with lower risk of mortality, especially for older people.[38] And in a study of more than twenty-two thousand people in the United Kingdom, people who were overweight but had healthy levels of blood cholesterol and other risk factors were no more likely to develop heart disease than were people who were slender.[39]

It's all the more reason to turn attention away from the scale and toward healthy habits.

DITCH THE DIET AND EMBRACE HEALTHY EATING

A big part of healthful eating is to choose healthy foods, of course. Another part is to develop a more "connected" eating style. This means eating when you are hungry and stopping when you are full. People who are used to following prescribed diets sometimes don't know how to do that. It's also a challenge if you often eat in response to emotions or other nonhunger cues. It can, in fact, take some time and practice to learn to hear those hunger and satiety signals.

Try this for your next few meals: Eat slowly, away from all distractions, paying attention to how the food tastes and how you feel. Stop eating when you are satisfied.

It's also helpful to experiment with "meal mixes" to see what kind of meal you find most satisfying and filling. Protein-rich meals often provide better satiety, and so do fiber-rich foods. That makes beans an especially good choice, as they are abundant in both. Many people find that including a little bit of fat in meals also helps to provide a feeling of satisfaction that keeps them full for a while.

Although it's important to keep the focus on healthful foods, make sure you include your favorite treats, too. A more restrained eating pattern—one that involves counting calories or that demonizes certain foods—can prevent you from learning to eat mindfully and intuitively. When you get too bogged down in rules, you might forget to pay attention to your body's signals. For good health, it's what you *usually* eat that matters. You may choose to limit or avoid certain foods based on your own preferences, but when any foods—oils, treats, veggie meats, or nuts and seeds—are viewed as "forbidden," it can trigger unhealthy views on food and fear-based food choices. Vegan meals should be pleasurable, not anxiety-producing!

No plant foods are off-limits with this approach, because a successful healthy eating plan is one that includes foods you enjoy, doesn't leave you feeling hungry or unsatisfied, and supports your health. You know, of course, that eating cupcakes all day long isn't going to do much good for your health. But this is where mindful eating comes in. If you are really listening to how you feel, you'll know that you don't feel great or satisfied when you just eat cupcakes.

Research shows that for those who have struggled for years with weight, an approach that focuses on healthy practices and mindful eating can build self-esteem and happiness, and improve overall health.[40] And a vegan diet is such a great fit to this approach. It automatically guides us toward choices that are more health promoting, and it reminds us that our food choices make a difference—for the environment, for animals, and for our own health—no matter what our body size is.

> "My body loves my vegan diet. I struggle with my weight as I have my entire life, but it is much easier to manage on a plant-based diet, especially as I eat primarily whole plant foods rather than processed foods (not always, but mostly). My skin, hair, and energy have all improved since I've been vegan. Overall I have never felt healthier and beyond my physical body, my spirit feels healthier. Veganism feeds my soul in a way that I did not expect; I feel a particular kind of joy and connectedness to the physical world and to my fellow creatures that I have never experienced before." —EMILY (51)

- Choose a variety of foods to meet nutritional needs, using the guidelines in this chapter.
- Eat intuitively, paying close attention to hunger and satiety signals.
- Find foods that satisfy your hunger and that you enjoy.
- Find an exercise program that you enjoy.
- Celebrate your veganism. It's a positive choice whether you lose weight or not.

HEALTHY VEGAN DIETS ARE EASY

Choosing a vegan diet that meets nutrient needs and protects your health is easy. When you fill your plate with fruits, vegetables, legumes, whole grains, nuts, and seeds; take supplements of vitamins B_{12} and D, and perhaps omega-3 fats; and give a little attention to calcium-rich foods, you won't have any problems getting enough of what your body needs.

But we can refine those choices a little bit to give extra protection against chronic diseases, such as heart disease, diabetes, and cancer. The next chapter will show you how you can get maximum benefit from your vegan diet.

VEGANS OVER 50 TELL THEIR STORIES

"I love being vegan." | Marisa Monagle

Marisa's story: "I am going to be fifty-five in September and my husband Bernie is fifty-seven. In August 2011, Bernie said to me he would like to eat more ethically. Unbeknownst to him I was doing a lot of thinking about going vegetarian; we were not huge meat eaters but we did eat meat. So I said, 'Let's just go vegetarian.' For him it was about the planet; for me it was about the animals."

Over the next five months, Marisa did some investigating online, where she met vegans through animal groups. She tried to watch the documentary *Earthlings* but lasted only five minutes. "Then when I watched a video on dairy farming. I told Bernie that we couldn't drink milk any more. We also stopped eating cheese."

For Marisa, being vegan is almost a spiritual journey. "I am not religious but it is as close as I will get. I feel that I can step on this earth with a clear conscience, knowing my living does not harm any animals. I love this. I have always loved animals and I am just sad that I didn't try harder earlier. But I am doing the right thing now."

Although Marisa's first blood tests showed she had low iron and B_{12} she turned that around within the year. "My eyes are so clear many people comment on this. I have not lost any weight but that could be due to sitting most days trying to finish a PhD! I do love my vegan sweet treats. I am sleeping better than ever, too, not going to bed with a stomach full of animal products."

Marisa and Bernie have turned their backyard into a rescue paradise for ten bunnies and a dog and soon will have four ex-battery hens. "Maybe in time we'll have some land and more animals.

"I have struggled with opening up my eyes to factory farming and have to work on not letting it get me too down. We live not too far from a slaughterhouse and I struggle when I pass cattle trucks. Bernie doesn't go out of his way to hear about stories of animal cruelty, as he can't handle those. But he is doing more than most people by being vegan.

"Our grown-up daughters think in their words we are 'f**kin hippies' but they are always happy to eat vegan food when at our home, and when we go out together.

"I love being vegan. It's the biggest most important thing I have ever done for the world and for me. There is no going back for us. I look forward to having grandchildren and teaching them to love animals and explaining why we don't eat meat, when they ask."

VEGAN DIETS FOR LIFELONG HEALTH

THE FOOD CHOICES described in Chapter 5 will go a long way toward reducing your risk for chronic conditions, such as heart disease, diabetes, and cancer.

Even among vegans, though, some dietary patterns are more protective than others. The guidelines for preventing chronic disease are simple, however, and they follow a one-diet-fits-all prescription based on slowly digested carbohydrates, healthy fats, abundant fruits and vegetables, and specific plant proteins that give vegans a unique edge.

NORMAL AGING IS DISEASE-FREE

Four types of chronic disease are so common among older Americans that we often think of them as normal consequences of aging. They aren't. While distinct changes—such as the ones we talked about in Chapter 4—are a part of normal aging, chronic diseases are not.

Cardiovascular disease, which includes high blood pressure, heart disease, and stroke, is strongly related to diet and lifestyle. And although there is a genetic predisposition for type 2 diabetes, much evidence suggests that this too is a disease that can often be prevented, and sometimes reversed, with a healthy diet and exercise program. The dietary connection to cancer and Alzheimer's disease isn't quite as clear—at least not yet. But, what we know about these diseases suggests that you can do much to lower your risk for both with a healthy vegan diet.

It's not to say that we know the diet that will make you disease-proof. Yes, genetics matter, and so do environmental factors that may be beyond your control. There is also the matter of your life history. The choices you made in the first twenty or thirty years of life (or that were made for you in childhood) can impact disease risk in your seventies and eighties. The truth is that we cannot guarantee good health. Sometimes, despite our best efforts and best choices, other factors beyond our control step in. But the idea is to control what we can, and diet is certainly one of those things.

Let's look first at how and why these diseases occur. You'll see that there are certain underlying similarities among all of them, and a number of ways in which food can play a role in risk reduction and treatment.

> *"At a family reunion a year and a half ago I was explaining my veganism to a cousin and that one reason I was vegan was for health reasons. She said, 'Why, are you sick?' People just don't understand about the preventative reasons for eating healthfully."* —CONNIE (52)

Research on Vegan Health

Most information about the health of vegans comes from just a handful of studies:

- The European Prospective Investigation into Cancer–Oxford (EPIC-Oxford) started in 1993 in the United Kingdom. It has examined the relationship of diet to chronic diseases, such as cancer and heart disease, in more than 65,000 subjects. More than one third of those subjects are vegetarians and around 2,500 are vegans.

■ The Adventist Health Study (AHS) was the only large-scale study for decades on the health of vegetarians in the United States. All of the subjects are members of the Seventh-day Adventist Church, living in California. Of the 34,192 subjects, 29 percent are vegetarian and around 7 percent, or around 2,400 people, are vegan. It has looked primarily at cancer and heart disease.

■ In 2002, the Adventist Health Study-2 (AHS-2) was started. Looking again at Seventh-day Adventists, it has a much larger study group—about 96,000 people—living in all fifty US states. Again, around 30 percent are vegetarians, and it also has a large population of vegans, more than 7,500 subjects. AHS-2 is already starting to provide useful information about vegan health.

■ Smaller studies from England, Germany, and the Slovak Republic have also produced findings about the health of vegans.

CARDIOVASCULAR DISEASE

Cardiovascular disease starts with damage to the endothelium, which is the smooth layer of cells lining the arteries. When the endothelium is damaged, cholesterol, fats, protein, and calcium can work their way into the artery, forming a plaque. Arteries become hard and narrow, the condition known as atherosclerosis, making it more difficult for blood to find its way to organs, including the heart and the brain. Heart disease occurs when the arteries to the heart are blocked. Cerebral vascular disease occurs when arteries to the brain are blocked, which can result in a stroke.

But arteries leading to other organs can also be affected. For example, cardiovascular disease is often related to erectile dysfunction, which affects more than 30 percent of men between the ages of forty and seventy. In fact, erectile dysfunction can be an early warning sign of atherosclerosis and impending heart disease.

Factors that cause damage to the endothelium include smoking and air pollution—both produce chemicals that assault the endothelial lining. Elevated blood cholesterol is especially damaging to the endothelium. In particular, LDL cholesterol (the bad cholesterol) is thought to be especially dangerous. It becomes harmful when it is oxidized, so oxidative stress also promotes atherosclerosis (see page 106).

HDL cholesterol (the good cholesterol), on the other hand, may help to protect against heart disease. It ferries excess cholesterol away from the arteries to the liver to be degraded and excreted. The extent of protection from HDLs isn't clear, although they may be more important for women than men, and may be especially important for people with diabetes.[1]

Other factors that promote atherosclerosis are high blood pressure, elevated triglycerides (fat molecules that circulate in the blood), high blood glucose, and extra fat around your middle.

Chronic inflammation is also an underlying cause of atherosclerosis. We think of inflammation as something that occurs around an injury, causing redness, swelling, and pain. In that case, inflammation is a short-term effect that is part of the immune system's healing process. It goes away when healing is achieved. Chronic inflammation is a more subtle version of that condition—you won't feel it—that persists and may cause damage to tissues throughout the body. It's thought to promote not just atherosclerosis but also diabetes and Alzheimer's disease. It may contribute to cancer, too. Factors that promote chronic inflammation include stress, smoking, oxidative stress, high blood glucose levels, and trans fats (see page 123 for more on trans fats).

Heart Disease

People who eat plant-based diets tend to have fewer risk factors for heart disease. Vegans in the United States and Europe typically have lower blood pressure,[2] and lower cholesterol levels.[3] People who eat a plant-based diet also have lower levels of inflammation and less oxidative stress.[4] This all suggests that vegans are at much lower risk for heart disease and stroke. It also suggests that a vegan diet might be a good way to treat these diseases.

The power of a plant-based diet in fighting heart disease was dramatically demonstrated back in 1990 at the California Pacific Medical Center. Dr. Dean Ornish and colleagues put study participants on a very low-fat vegetarian diet as part of a comprehensive lifestyle program that also emphasized exercise and stress management and provided social support. The diet wasn't vegan but was close to it. Many of the subjects who stuck with the program didn't just stop the progression of their heart disease; they appeared to have small reductions in the amount of plaque in their arteries. In comparison, most of the subjects who followed a more standard cholesterol-lowering plan actually got worse.

Although diet was just one part of this program—so we can't say how much of the benefit came directly from food choices—other studies looking at vegan diets have found them to be very beneficial. Researchers from the University of Toronto investigated the effects of a high-fat, high-protein vegan diet on blood cholesterol levels—an approach they dubbed the Eco-Atkins diet.

In this study, twenty-two people followed the diet for four weeks, getting their protein from seitan, soy, vegetables, nuts, and grains, and their fat from nuts, vegetable oils, and soy foods. They experienced reductions in their LDL cholesterol and ended up with better cholesterol profiles than did subjects who followed a low-fat, high-carbohydrate, almost-vegan diet. The Eco-Atkins group also rated their diet as more satiating compared to the people eating the high-carb diet.[5]

These studies tell us that different types of vegan diets can be very effective in fighting heart disease.

DIABETES

When you eat potatoes, bread, bananas, or any carb-rich food, the carbohydrate (starch) molecules are broken down to their individual building blocks of glucose. As the glucose passes from the intestines into the blood, the pancreas pumps out insulin, a hormone needed to escort glucose into the cells. Because glucose serves as the cells' main source of fuel, getting it into cells is crucial for survival.

In diabetes, there are problems with the way the body uses or produces insulin. In type 1 diabetes (which used to be called juvenile diabetes), the pancreas produces too little insulin or none at all. People with type 1 diabetes need to take injections of insulin, or deliver insulin by pump. This type of diabetes is thought to be an autoimmune condition. Before the discovery of insulin it was a death sentence; now it can be well controlled with insulin and diet.

Type 2 diabetes is much more common and is a disease of insulin resistance: cells become resistant to the effects of insulin and won't absorb glucose. Insulin resistance is a response to high blood levels of insulin. Frequent consumption of quickly digested carbohydrates can cause repeated spikes in blood glucose, followed by surges in insulin production. Over time, cells may react by ignoring the insulin. The result is chronically elevated levels of blood glucose, which can damage arteries and cause other health problems.

Type 2 diabetes appears to be the result of both genetics and lifestyle. That is, some people are at higher risk for type 2 diabetes because of their genes or genetic makeup, but it can still often be prevented by healthy lifestyle. It's another condition where extra fat around your middle can raise risk, and so can inflammation.

Both types of diabetes raise risk for a number of health problems, including heart disease and dementia. So it's important to control blood glucose levels and to also eat in a way that lowers blood cholesterol and protects the health of the arteries.

While it might seem that high-carb diets promote the glucose and insulin surges that can lead to insulin resistance, this doesn't seem to be true. In fact, vegetarians typically eat more carbohydrates than meat eaters do, but still tend to have less insulin resistance compared to omnivores. That is, they are more "insulin sensitive."[6]

This is probably because vegetarians consume more fiber and tend to favor foods like legumes and whole grains that are digested and absorbed more slowly, causing gentler elevations in insulin. Their better insulin sensitivity may translate to protection from diabetes, especially for vegans. Researchers from Loma Linda University compared rates of type 2 diabetes in more than sixty thousand participants in the Adventist Health Study-2. Vegans were about half as likely as meat eaters to have diabetes. In fact, they were less likely to have diabetes than were even lacto-ovo vegetarians.[7]

Vegan and near-vegan diets can be used to treat diabetes. As is true for the diets used to treat atherosclerosis, both low-fat and high-fat diets are effective as long as they are based on whole plant foods. Researchers associated with the Physicians Committee for Responsible Medicine (PCRM) tested the effects of a very low-fat diet for control of diabetes. They asked study participants to avoid all animal products and fatty foods and to favor slowly digested, carbohydrate-rich foods, such as beans. Not only was the diet effective at controlling blood glucose levels, but many participants thought it was easier to follow than a more traditional diet used to treat diabetes. The fact that they didn't need to measure foods or restrict amounts made the diet especially appealing.[8]

Researchers in the Czech Republic used a somewhat different almost-vegan approach (just one serving daily of dairy foods and no other animal products) to manage diabetes. This diet was considerably higher in fat than was the PCRM diet, but was calorie reduced. When compared to a standard diet used to treat diabetes, the near-vegan diet was more effective in controlling blood glucose levels and eliminating medication used to treat diabetes.[9]

CANCER

Cancer occurs when abnormal cells divide and replicate in an uncontrolled manner. Under normal circumstances, the cells of your body grow and divide in an orderly and tightly controlled fashion, passing along perfect copies of your DNA as new cells are needed to keep the body healthy. If DNA becomes damaged or changed in some way, however, the result can be cells that don't respond to normal controls. Wayward cell growth and reproduction can lead to tumor growth. Over time and many mutations (damage to DNA), the tumor itself can acquire the ability to invade nearby tissues and the cancer cells can travel to other parts of the body through the blood and lymph.

There are many stages to the process, occurring over years and even decades. The body has its own repair systems for damaged DNA, so most of the damage that occurs never goes on to cause a problem. It takes a lot of mistakes over a long period of time for most cancers to gain a foothold in the body. And there are many opportunities to stop the cancer from ever developing or to keep it from progressing. For example, dietary antioxidants can prevent initial damage to DNA, stopping the cancer process in its tracks. Other phytochemicals in plant foods may inhibit the ability of tumors to spread to adjacent organs. Still others inhibit formation of the blood vessels that tumors need for growth.

People who have inherited mutations on certain "cancer genes" are at higher risk for certain cancers. The best known of these are the breast cancer genes BRCA-1 and BRCA-2 that are most common among Jewish women of Eastern European ancestry. Other cancer genes are important, too. It's possible that a healthy diet can prevent genes from being "expressed," although we have limited research on this.[10]

Studying Diet and Cancer

Measuring the effects of diet on heart disease risk or hypertension is easy. Researchers gather together a group of study participants, feed them several different diets, and watch what happens to their blood cholesterol, blood pressure, or even their weight.

Studying cancer is trickier, because it's a disease with fewer well-accepted markers of risk and it develops over a long period of time. As a result, we often depend on epidemiologic studies—the type of study that follows large groups of people for many years, tracks what they eat and looks for links between diet and disease. These studies are harder to control and they show associations, not cause and effect.

So, while we have some good ideas about what type of diets reduce or raise the risk for cancer, the evidence is not as strong as we'd like it to be. What we know does suggest that the kind of diet that lowers risk for heart disease and hypertension is most likely also going to help protect you from cancer—that is, a diet that focuses on plants appears to be protective.

Studying cancer in vegans brings some additional challenges, however. Most studies lump vegans and lacto-ovo vegetarians together, making it hard to determine whether one group has more or less protection than the other. And many of the people in these studies who say they are vegetarian actually eat some meat or fish.[11] (This is a big problem in vegetarian research.) The little bit of research we have on vegan cancer rates is encouraging, though. In the Adventist Health Study-2, vegans had lower rates of cancer than did either meat eaters or lacto-ovo vegetarians, and this was especially true for cancers specific to women.[12]

ALZHEIMER'S DISEASE AND DEMENTIA

The memory lapses that come a little more frequently as years go by are annoying. But true dementia—which is a disease, not a normal consequence of aging—is devastating.

Alzheimer's disease (AD) is the most common type of dementia, affecting memory, judgment, verbal ability, and personality over time. It's characterized by tissue degeneration that produces beta-amyloids—deposits of plaque—in the brain. They're made of protein fragments that are normally broken down and discarded in the healthy brain. In Alzheimer's disease, they accumulate and form into hard deposits. The other hallmark of AD is the accumulation of abnormal tangles of a protein called tau. Again, the presence of tau in the brain is normal. It's the twisted tangles that are not.

AD has a genetic component, but there is also growing evidence that lifestyle can greatly reduce your risk of ever getting this type of dementia. Insulin resistance, high blood cholesterol, oxidative stress, and chronic inflammation are all linked to a higher risk for AD.[13]

Another type of dementia is multi-infarct dementia. It occurs when atherosclerosis causes arteries leading to the brain to narrow, reducing the flow of oxygen to brain cells. This can result in a succession of small strokes that go unnoticed but do damage to brain cells, leading over time to dementia. Keeping both blood cholesterol and blood pressure low, exercising, and avoiding smoking can all go a long way toward preventing multi-infarct or vascular dementia.

We don't know whether vegans have a lower risk for AD or multi-infarct dementia because those studies haven't been done. But we do know that vegans have lower cholesterol, less hypertension, and probably less inflammation. It seems pretty clear that a plant-based diet is a good place to start for preventing dementia.

"I am one of the few men of my age that I know who are on no medications—I feel quite left out when they discuss their lipitor and warfarin."—DES (61)

HOW VEGAN DIETS PROTECT AGAINST CHRONIC DISEASE

Although the chronic diseases that plague so many Americans all appear to be unique, they are all related through common underlying causes—inflammation, oxidative stress, and insulin resistance. (See Table 3-1 for a quick review of these conditions.) Trading in usual Western eating practices for a diet based on more whole plant foods is an important part of a lifestyle approach to preventing these conditions and the chronic diseases they promote. We've already seen that vegan and near-vegan diets can be useful for treating these diseases, too.

The vegan and near-vegan diets used to reverse and control heart disease and diabetes have all been slightly different, but they share some important similarities. All are based on whole plant foods, using minimal amounts of processed foods, and they are either very low in fat or include healthy plant fats. And they are, of course, either devoid of animal foods or include only very small amounts. The evidence suggests that a variety of factors contribute to the healthful effects of these diets. Some benefits come from certain components of plant foods. Others come from the absence of harmful compounds in animal foods.

TABLE 3-1: DIVERSE CONDITIONS, COMMON CAUSES: INFLAMMATION, OXIDATIVE STRESS, AND INSULIN RESISTANCE

	RAISES RISK FOR THESE DISEASES	PREVENTED BY
Chronic inflammation: Systemic inflammation throughout the body	Heart disease, diabetes, cancer, Alzheimer's disease, rheumatoid arthritis	Exercise, slowly digested carbs, stress management, maybe long-chain omega-3 fats DHA and EPA, other healthy fats
Oxidative stress: An imbalance between the free radicals that promote oxidation and the antioxidant systems that neutralize it	Skin aging, muscle loss, dementia, heart disease, cancer, osteoarthritis	Antioxidant-rich diet (whole-plant foods, especially fruits and vegetables), sun protection, avoidance of tobacco, slowly digested carbs
Insulin resistance: A condition characterized by high blood levels of glucose and insulin. Cells become resistant to the effects of insulin and won't take up glucose from blood.	Diabetes, heart disease, cancer, Alzheimer's disease	Slowly digested carbs, exercise

HAZARDS FROM ANIMAL FOODS

Good things happen as soon as you remove meat, dairy, and eggs from your plate. Your diet automatically becomes cholesterol-free because there is never any cholesterol in plants. More important, your intake of saturated fat drops, too.

Saturated fat raises blood cholesterol levels, promoting damage to arteries and raising risk for atherosclerosis. Saturated fat may also be linked to Alzheimer's disease, insulin resistance, and some types of cancer.[14] Dietary cholesterol has a lesser effect on heart disease risk, but may raise risk for some cancers.[15]

A vegan diet more or less guarantees that you will be eating foods low in saturated fat. In the EPIC-Oxford study, vegans consumed less than half the saturated fat of omnivores. With a few exceptions—such as coconut oil and chocolate—plant foods contain only small amounts of saturated fat. Most of the saturated fat in American diets comes from meat, cheese, milk, butter, and eggs, all of which are abundant in it. And all of the cholesterol in nonvegan diets comes from animal foods, as there is none in plants.

Meat is also high in iron. And while that may sound like a good thing, there may be a downside to getting too much of this essential nutrient. Younger women lose iron every month through menstruation, which protects them from iron overload. But men and postmenopausal women have no way to get rid of excess iron except for small amounts lost through sweat and when intestinal cells slough off.

One concern is that iron accumulates in the brain of people with AD.[16] We don't know whether this contributes to dementia or is a consequence of unhealthy brain tissue, but it may be worth protecting against excessive iron levels to lower risk for dementia.

Iron is a pro-oxidant—a compound that promotes oxidation. It's possible that it raises risk for heart disease for this reason. Although this is a theory that is falling out of favor a little bit, some evidence points to a harmful effect of high iron stores for heart health of women especially.[17]

Although plant foods are actually very high in iron, it is in a different form than the kind found in animal foods. The iron in plant foods is often bound to compounds called phytates, which makes the iron harder to absorb. We can get enough iron from these foods but are at a much lower risk of getting too much. The iron in red meats and poultry, on the other hand, is always well absorbed, so people who eat these foods can end up with high levels of iron in their body.

Finally, dairy consumption is linked to higher levels of a compound called insulin-like growth factor-1 (IGF-1), which may promote cancer.[18] In the EPIC-Oxford study, IGF-1 levels were 9 percent lower in vegan men compared to both meat eaters and vegetarians.[19] There is also evidence that men who consume lots of dairy foods are at higher risk for prostate cancer.[20]

Red Meat, White Meat, or No Meat?

One of the strongest dietary links to cancer risk involves red meat, primarily beef. Diets high in red meat raise risk for colon cancer in particular, but other cancers as well. And of course, red meat is also high in the saturated fat, which may contribute to heart disease and Alzheimer's disease. A study at the Cleveland Clinic has suggested that another compound found in red meat, carnitine, is metabolized by meat eaters to produce a compound called TMAO that contributes to atherosclerosis. That would mean that even lean cuts of red meat that are lower in saturated fat could still raise your risk for having a heart attack.

Whether carnitine is harmful may depend upon the type of bacteria you have in your intestine. Vegans host different types of bacteria in their colons, and interestingly, according to the Cleveland Clinic study, they didn't produce TMAO when, for the sake of science, they ate meat.[21]

For many people, a seemingly obvious solution has been to cut way back on their red meat intake, replacing it with chicken and turkey. It's true that these foods are often lower in both saturated fat and carnitine, and they have not been linked nearly as strongly to cancer risk or heart disease. You'll see below, when we talk about health benefits associated with plant foods, that replacing one kind of animal food with another is not really the best route to better health. But it's certainly true that lower-fat meat from chickens and fish is less damaging to your health than red meat.

The problem is that eating these less harmful meats ends up causing greater harm to animals. Some of the worst and cruelest practices on farms involve chickens and turkeys. Even on "free-range" and organic farms, and on most "family" farms, these animals are raised under conditions of extreme confinement and conditions that are often painful and distressing. And while the slaughterhouse is awful for any animal, it's worst of all for birds. They are exempt from the Humane Slaughter Act, which means that there are no laws regarding the way they are treated and killed. And because chickens are small, eating even 4 ounces of their meat twice per week translates to the death of as many as a dozen birds each year.

It's a dilemma—eating chicken and turkey might be (somewhat) better for you than eating cows and pigs, but it inflicts even more suffering on animals. And, of course, it's equally harmful to the environment. That's why a vegan diet is truly the only option for those who want to eat in a way that translates to optimal health and compassion for animals.

THE POWER OF PLANTS

Ditching animal products isn't just about losing the bad stuff in those foods. What you'll gain is every bit as important. Vegan diets are almost always higher in a wide range of factors and compounds that protect health and reduce risk for chronic disease. But you won't reduce your chronic disease risk if you swap out steak for white rice and doughnuts. Loading up your plate with refined carbs is just as bad as piling it with steak, eggs, and cheese. So while adding more plant foods to your diet is a great first step toward reducing chronic disease risk, you'll want to maximize the benefits by choosing antioxidant-rich foods, healthy fats, and slowly digested carbohydrates.

Antioxidants Fight Chronic Disease

We saw in Chapter 5 that oxidative stress contributes to aging. It may also be a driving factor in atherosclerosis, cancer, diabetes, and dementia. Animal foods contain antioxidants, but their content pales in comparison to plant foods which have as much as sixty-four times more antioxidant activity.[22] The antioxidants in plants include vitamins—such as C and E—as well as thousands of phytochemicals.

All plant foods provide antioxidants, but fruits and vegetables are antioxidant powerhouses. This may help explain why, in a study of more than 300,000 people from eight European countries, people who ate at least eight servings of fruits and vegetables per day were 22 percent less likely to have heart disease than were those who ate fewer than three servings.[23]

Herbs and spices are also wonderful sources of antioxidants—so dressing up your meals with these natural flavors is a good way to sneak more antioxidants into your diet.

Although many of the phytochemicals in fruits and vegetables are antioxidants, some act in other ways to protect health. For example, compounds in citrus fruits induce enzyme systems that detoxify carcinogens in the body. Compounds in berries can act as antioxidants while also disrupting formation of blood vessels that feed tumors.

Food preparation can have a big effect on the protective effect of compounds in vegetables. Take lycopene, for example, an antioxidant in tomatoes that has been linked to reduced risk for prostate cancer.[24] It's absorbed much better from cooked and processed tomato products, such as tomato sauce. So, eating raw tomatoes won't give you the same robust protection as would a bowl of pasta with marinara sauce.[25]

In contrast, compounds called glucosinolates, which may reduce risk for cancer and which are abundant in members of the cabbage family, are absorbed best from raw vegetables.

This isn't something you need to micromanage—it's fine to eat raw tomatoes and cooked Brussels sprouts. But the findings show that both raw and cooked vegetables are important in healthy vegan diets.

Good Carbs: Fiber and Resistant Starch

It's not surprising that vegans and vegetarians have much higher fiber intakes than meat eaters do because fiber is found only in plant foods. Whole grains, beans, nuts, seeds, fruits, and vegetables are all abundant in fiber. Refined grains don't have much, and meat, dairy, and eggs have none.

Fiber may help with weight control and also lowers risk for colon cancer and heart disease. In women high-fiber diets are linked to lower estrogen levels, which may in turn protect against breast cancer.[26]

Fiber also slows the absorption of glucose into the bloodstream, which keeps levels of both glucose and insulin more even and sustained. This helps prevent the insulin resistance that is a precursor to diabetes. Soluble fiber, the type that is abundant in dry beans, sweet potatoes, oats and barley, is especially beneficial for lowering blood cholesterol levels.

Plants also contain resistant starch—starch that is resistant to digestive enzymes. It's metabolized in the colon by bacteria, producing compounds that may improve satiety and help to lower blood cholesterol. This may explain why vegetarians have more beneficial types of bacteria in their colon, the kind that may protect against colon cancer.[27] Good sources of resistant starch include uncooked oats, bananas, beans, pasta, and rye or pumpernickel bread.[28]

In contrast to foods that are packed with fiber and resistant starch, refined carbs dump glucose into the blood, causing a rapid increase in both blood glucose and insulin. These in turn raise the risk of insulin resistance, which promotes heart disease, diabetes, and maybe cancer.

It's okay to enjoy some warm bread at your favorite Italian restaurant or a slice of cake for dessert, as long as the foods at the center of your diet are whole, unrefined ones. And for your carb-rich choices, aim to eat more of the ones that are rich in soluble fiber and/or resistant starch: barley, oats, pasta, beans, sweet potatoes, and rye or pumpernickel bread.

PAINLESS AGING

COULD A VEGAN DIET benefit people who suffer from painful conditions, such as rheumatoid arthritis and osteoarthritis? It might.

Rheumatoid arthritis is an autoimmune disease that causes inflammation, pain, and stiffness in the joints and their surrounding tissues. People with rheumatoid arthritis are also at higher risk for heart disease.

Any diet that reduces chronic inflammation might help to relieve symptoms of rheumatoid arthritis. A vegan diet that is low in saturated fat and rich in slowly digested carbohydrates and antioxidant-rich foods is a good place to start for reduction of symptoms. The long- chain omega-3 fats DHA and EPA have anti-inflammatory properties, too, so taking algae-derived supplements of these fats could be a good idea.

Osteoarthritis is a result of the wear and tear on joints that comes with age. This causes cartilage, the tissue that cushions bones at the joints, to break down. Oxidative stress can promote cartilage breakdown, which suggests some benefits for vegans, as we have fewer markers of oxidative stress in our blood.[29] A couple of vegan supplements also appear to help with symptoms of osteoarthritis. These are extracts of soybean and avocado oils, called avocado/soybean unsaponifiables (ASUs), and glucosamine sulfate.[30]

Healthy Fats

A drizzle of olive oil over a salad or a sprinkle of dark sesame oil in stir-fried vegetables can make all the difference to the flavor and appeal of a dish. That's different from the way most Americans eat, though. We're used to dishes that are swimming in fats and oils.

Fatty meals can drive up your calorie intake, take a toll on the health of your arteries, and displace other nutritious foods in meals. A single high-fat meal, such as one you might find at a fast-food restaurant, can do acute damage to the endothelial lining of the arteries. This doesn't mean that you need to cut fat out of your diet, though. The healthiest populations in the world use added fats in their plant-based menus: olive oil along the Mediterranean, peanut and sesame oil in Asia, and coconut oil in parts of southeast Asia. Their menus are fundamentally different from the fatty, disease-promoting diet so common in the United States. They are diets that are based on whole plant foods and that use mostly healthy fats.

Polyunsaturated fats in vegetable oils, nuts and seeds lower blood cholesterol when they replace saturated fat in meals. Foods rich in monounsaturated fats, such as almonds and hazelnuts, and olive and canola oils, may have health benefits, too.

Depending on genetics, restricting fat too much can backfire. In some people, very low-fat diets produce LDL-cholesterol particles that are small and dense. This makes it easier for the cholesterol to penetrate artery walls. Diets that include healthy plant fats, on the other hand, produce larger more buoyant LDL-cholesterol particles that are far less harmful.[31]

Some people with diabetes find it easier to control blood glucose levels when they replace some of the carbohydrate in their diets with healthy fats.[32]

Plant fats may also benefit men who have had prostate cancer. The Health Professionals Follow-up Study started in 1986 with more than 50,000 male health professionals to assess relationships between diet and health in older men. A recent analysis of 4,600 of these subjects who had been diagnosed with prostate cancer looked at the link between the men's postdiagnosis diet and rates of survival. Men who replaced 10 percent of the calories from carbohydrates in their diet with fat from vegetable oils and nuts were 29 percent less likely to die from prostate cancer and 26 percent less likely to die from other causes.[33]

HEALTHY FATS FROM NUTS: Nuts are high-fat foods that especially deserve a place on your plate. When researchers from Loma Linda University teamed up with researchers from Barcelona to analyze twenty-five studies of nuts and cholesterol levels, they found that eating about 2.5 ounces of nuts per day—a little more than ½ cup—

could lower LDL cholesterol by 7.5 percent. Eating nuts also lowered triglyceride levels.[34]

That's impressive enough on its own. But when researchers looked at the relationship of nuts to actual rates of heart disease, they found that these foods decreased risk substantially—to a much greater extent than what those cholesterol reductions could explain.[35] This means that there is more to nuts than their effect on blood cholesterol levels. Part of their protection may come from their high content of arginine, an amino acid that converts to a compound (nitric oxide) that helps to keep blood vessels relaxed.[36] Consuming nuts and vegetable oils can also reduce inflammation and oxidative stress.[37]

And while it seems counterintuitive, including some nuts in your diet could even help with weight management. The old-fashioned idea about fat and weight loss was that they can't go together. It made sense, as every gram of fat has more than twice as many calories as a gram of protein or carbohydrate. But including a little bit of fat in diets sometimes produces a feeling of satisfaction and satiety that makes it easier to cut back on calories. Furthermore, evidence suggests that we don't absorb all of the calories from nuts and that they can give your metabolism a little boost.[38] (This doesn't apply to nut butters, only to whole nuts.) Even so, snacking on nuts all day will push your calorie intake up too high. In contrast, eating a serving or two—¼ to ½ cup—of whole nuts per day may actually make it easier to eat less food overall.

INCLUDING HIGHER-FAT FOODS IN HEALTHY VEGAN DIETS: The health benefits of higher-fat plant foods were not as well recognized several decades ago, when very low-fat eating patterns first became popular. But as research has evolved in the past twenty years regarding plant fats and health, so have dietary recommendations. On its nutrition website, the Harvard School of Public Health recently said this about dietary fats: "It's time to end the low-fat myth.[. . .] 'Good' fats—monounsaturated and polyunsaturated fats—lower disease risk. 'Bad' fats—saturated and, especially, trans fats—increase disease risk."

So don't be afraid to include nuts, seeds, or healthy vegetable oils in your diet. Even if you prefer lower-fat meals, when these foods are used condiment style—nuts sprinkled over a salad or a few teaspoons of oil used to sauté vegetables—they are a good fit to healthy vegan eating.

TRANS FATS

NOT ALL FATS IN vegan foods are benign. Trans fats are produced when hydrogen is added to vegetable oils to produce a solid fat that won't get rancid. Trans fats raise LDL cholesterol and lower HDL-cholesterol levels, and they promote inflammation.[39] Even small intakes of these fats may raise risk for disease. It's easy to avoid them, though. They are found mostly in highly processed snack foods, such as chips and baked goods. Although trans fat content must be listed on the Nutrition Facts panel of food labels, any food that contains less than 0.5 gram of trans fat can claim "0 grams of trans fat." Those small amounts can add up to provide too much trans fat in your diet. To avoid these fats completely, look for the phrase "partially hydrogenated oil" on the label. Those words signal to you that the product contains trans fats and should be avoided or greatly minimized in your diet.

When cooking with oils, choose extra virgin olive oil over plain olive oil. It comes from the first press of the olives and is richer in the phytochemicals that may have disease-fighting properties. For salad dressings, try walnut oil, which provides the essential fatty acid ALA along with a wonderful savory flavor. Toasted sesame oil also adds exceptional flavor to Asian-style noodle dishes or stir-fried vegetables.

Look for cold-pressed oils because they are less processed and retain more of their phytochemicals. They are best for low-to-moderate-temperature cooking, such as a quick sauté over low heat, and are ideal for salad dressings. Store them in the refrigerator to keep them fresh. (Extra virgin olive oil doesn't need to be refrigerated.)

When you choose good-quality oils and use flavorful ones, such as extra virgin olive oil, walnut oil, and toasted sesame oil, you'll find that a little goes a long way.

Soy Protects Against Cancer and Heart Disease

Soybeans, first domesticated in northern China, have been part of Asian meals for centuries. Over the years, cooks learned to process these beans into some of the most important ingredients of Asian menus: tofu, soy milk, tempeh, and miso.

Soybeans are unique because they are the only commonly consumed food that provides substantial amounts of isoflavones. These are the plant estrogens that help to alleviate hot flashes in menopausal women. But their effects on health extend to possible protection against chronic disease.

Even though isoflavones are phytoestrogens, or plant estrogens, they are actually profoundly different from the female hormone estrogen. Their effects vary greatly throughout the body. They seem to have estrogen-like effects that lower hot flashes and build collagen, which reduces skin wrinkling.[40] But research suggests that, in other parts of the body, they don't mimic estrogen in any way. For example, estrogen is highly protective of bone health in women, but isoflavones don't seem to offer the same benefit. And while estrogen may promote breast cancer, isoflavones clearly don't.

In fact, early research on isoflavones was hopeful that they might actually lower risk for breast cancer. Current thinking is that isoflavones are in fact protective against breast cancer but only when they are consumed during childhood or adolescence.[41]

On the other hand, recent research has revealed that soy might offer some protection for women who have already had breast cancer. Studies in both China and the United States have found that women who consume the most soy have a better prognosis after a breast cancer diagnosis.[42] One analysis of nearly ten thousand breast cancer survivors found that higher soy intake was associated with a 17 percent reduction in death from breast cancer and a 25 percent reduction in tumor recurrence.[43]

Soy consumption may also help to explain the lower rates of prostate cancer among men in Asian countries. While men in China and Japan are just as likely as Western men to have prostate tumors, their tumors are far less likely to become life threatening. It's possible that the isoflavones in soy slow the growth of life-threatning prostate cancer cells. It could explain why Asian men with the highest soy intakes are only about half as likely to develop prostate cancer compared to those who seldom eat soyfoods.[44] In men who have been unsuccessfully treated for prostate cancer, several studies (although not all) found consumption of soy isoflavones slowed the rise in PSA levels, a marker of cancer progression.[45]

Soy reduces risk for heart disease, too. Isoflavones help arteries stay flexible and relaxed.[46] And it seems that even the protein in soy foods has benefits for heart health. Adding soy protein to the diet, if used to replace meat and dairy foods even without otherwise changing the saturated fat content of the diet, can help reduce LDL-cholesterol levels. It's a smallish effect, but the additive effects of soy—lower saturated fat, relaxation of endothelial lining, and cholesterol-suppressing effects of soy protein—can add up to a considerable impact. Among people in Japan and China, those who eat at least two servings of soy foods per day have half the risk for heart disease of those who consume only small amounts of soy.[47]

Note that though veggie meats and cheeses made from soy protein can be fun and easy ways to move away from meat and dairy foods, they can be low in isoflavones, which are often stripped away from the soybean when these foods are made. On the other hand, these convenience foods can be a great way to give your soy protein intake a boost. So it's fine to include these foods in your diet if you like them, but keep the focus on traditional soy foods, such as tofu, tempeh, edamame, soy milk, and miso.

POTASSIUM PROTECTS AGAINST CHRONIC DISEASE

POTASSIUM PROTECTS BONE HEALTH and lowers risk for hypertension and heart disease. Most Americans fall far short of the RDA for potassium, which is 4,700 milligrams per day. Some vegans don't get enough, either, but we tend to do a little better than the average meat eater. Legumes are especially rich in potassium, so replacing meat in meals with beans automatically gives your potassium intake a big boost. Make sure you eat plenty of potassium-rich foods every day. In addition to beans, the best sources are beet greens, spinach, sweet potatoes, Swiss chard, tomato juice, tomato sauce, V8 Juice, sea vegetables, bananas, and orange juice.

How Much Alcohol?

Alcohol has long been a regular part of many healthy cultural diets. In particular, red wine plays an important culinary role in the diets of Southern Europeans. Alcohol helps to maintain higher levels of the good HDL cholesterol that may protect against heart disease. Moderate amounts of alcohol are also associated with lower risk for diabetes and lower rates of inflammation[48] as well as better insulin sensitivity.[49] On the other hand, even moderate drinking raises the risk for breast cancer. Alcohol also takes a toll on bone health, and of course, too much of it will tax your liver.

If you don't drink, there is no reason to start just to reap the benefits we just discussed. There are plenty of other good things in vegan diets that will give you those same benefits. If you drink, limit yourself to one to two drinks per day and choose red wine or dark beer to get the advantages of their antioxidant content. Vegan women may have a particular advantage in that their diets are usually high in folate, which may mitigate some of the effects of alcohol consumption on breast cancer risk.[50]

Limit Sodium

Diets high in sodium are linked to hypertension, higher risk for heart disease and stroke, and also risk for osteoporosis. You don't need to go salt-free, but most people could stand to cut back on their sodium intake, and vegans are no exception. Foods that pile on the salt include most veggie meats and veggie cheeses, canned foods, snack chips and crackers, prepared vegetable stocks, and condiments, such as ketchup, mustard, miso and salsa. Whole plant foods are naturally low in sodium, so if you minimize your intake of processed foods, you'll automatically reduce your sodium intake. It's fine to include some processed foods in your diet when it's fun or convenient to do so. Just don't make them the center of your menus. And it's also okay to lightly salt your own home-cooked recipes. In particular, iodized salt can help vegans meet needs for the essential mineral iodine. If you prefer to use sea salt, make sure it's iodized.

Some vegans prefer to add salty flavors to their food by using tamari, which is a more authentic Japanese version of soy sauce. Although it is still a high-sodium food, tamari has a richer flavor, so you may find that you need less of it to flavor foods.

HEALTHY VEGAN DIETS IN A NUTSHELL

We can pull the information from this chapter and Chapter 5 into seven simple guidelines that will ensure that you meet nutrient needs and that will also maximize the disease-fighting benefits of your vegan diet.

1. **Pile your plate with fruits and vegetables.** They are packed with antioxidants that protect bone and muscle strength, protect eyesight, slow skin aging, keep your brain sharp, and lower the risk for heart disease, diabetes, and cancer. Many are good sources of potassium, which helps keep bones healthy and blood pressure in check.

2. **Take appropriate supplements.** Vitamin B_{12} keeps your blood and nervous system healthy. It protects cognitive function and reduces risk for heart disease. Vitamin D is important for bone health and may reduce risk for some chronic disease.

3. **Eat plenty of protein-rich foods such as beans and soy foods.** Protein protects your bones and muscles. The resistant starch and fiber in beans keeps blood glucose levels more even, lowering the risk for heart disease and diabetes. The isoflavones in soy may help prevent prostate cancer and protect the health of women who have had breast cancer. The protein in soy can lower blood cholesterol levels. The best sources are traditional soy foods, such as tofu, tempeh, soy milk, and edamame. It's fine to include veggie meats in your diet, though.

4. **Include good sources of calcium in your diet every day.** Foods that are rich in calcium include tofu, calcium-fortified plant-based milks and juices, kale, collards, turnip greens, bok choy, almond butter, sesame tahini, and figs.

5. **Choose carb-rich foods that are packed with resistant starch and fiber.** These help with weight control, prevent insulin resistance, lower cholesterol levels, and help prevent cancer. All grains and starchy vegetables are good choices. The best choices are barley, oats, pumpernickel and rye breads, pasta, and beans.

6. **Include healthy fats in your diet.** Fats from plants reduce blood cholesterol levels, inflammation, and oxidative stress. Meet your needs for the essential omega-3 fats with a small daily serving of ground flaxseeds, hemp seeds, walnuts, or chia seeds, or canola, walnut, or soy oil (see page 82). Nuts and seeds provide important nutrients like zinc and are linked to easier weight control, better management of blood glucose for people with diabetes, and protection from heart disease. Use vegetable oils in moderation to add flavor and texture to recipes. Consider supplementing your diet with a vegan source of DHA and EPA from algae.

7. **Keep alcohol and sodium intake moderate.** Men should limit alcohol to no more than two drinks per day. For women, it's best to limit intake to one drink per day. Keep sodium intake low by limiting processed foods.

What's in Our Fridges

Patti: There is usually soy milk in my fridge, and I try to buy those that are supplemented with vitamin D and calcium. Also, jars of pearled barley, quinoa, and rice are in there so as to keep kitchen bugs from feasting on them. You will probably find a few loaves of sourdough or sprouted bread in my freezer (I like Alvarado Street and Ezekiel brands). I am never without a few onions, a bunch of celery, and a bag of carrots, so I can make a soup in a hurry. There is usually at least one bunch of kale or collards, and broccoli or bok choy, too. I also keep dark and light miso in the fridge, plus a jar of prepared Dijon mustard, one of peanut butter, and one of sesame tahini. (A mixture of equal parts tahini and miso, plus a little water, makes one of my favorite salad dressings.) You might find Smart Bacon waiting to be made into a BLT, or Tofurky spicy turkey slices waiting to be sliced and added to a salad. I also love smoked tofu and buy a local brand called Tofu Yu at my supermarket. And my pantry almost always has red lentils, brown lentils, and canned beans of every variety. Garlic is always on the counter in a ceramic bowl, too.

Carol: My refrigerator always has some almond milk in it. If it's nighttime, you'll find my bowl of Refrigerator Oatmeal (see page 242) with a mixture of almond and flax milks softening it for the morning. There is always fruit in the fridge: blueberries for sure, and if I am lucky, raspberries or organic strawberries (it is thought that strawberries absorb pesticides, so I always choose organic ones at the store). My sesame tahini is there, as well as several different kinds of miso (I use red miso instead of Parmesan in pesto). Kale in some form is there: either a bunch of kale waiting to be prepared, or some leftover kale. I like to dip baby romaine lettuce in hummus, or stick it on sandwiches, so you'll find that as well. My seeds and nuts are kept in the refrigerator, too. At the beginning of the week, there may be a full container of soup, made over the weekend, and a quinoa/rice mix ready to be the base for a meal. Some days, you'll find tofu being pressed, so that it's ready to be baked or used in a tofu scramble. I always keep some store-bought vegan cheese just in case I crave a grilled cheese sandwich. It doesn't happen often, but when it does, I don't want to be thwarted! And finally, my favorite treat is toasting a vegan marshmallow, so a container of them is usually lingering in my fridge.

Ginny: I do bulk cooking every weekend, cooking whole grains and beans, cutting up salad ingredients, and making a few sauces to pull everything together. I love when my refrigerator is packed with these healthy foods plus a good selection of condiments and a few convenience items. It means that easy, satisfying meals are within reach at all times.

Peek inside my fridge and you'll almost always find quinoa (usually mixed with corn and onions) or brown rice or baked sweet potatoes, plus a big pot of lentil soup, and at least one other kind of bean dish. The little drawer that some people use for meat is packed with tofu, tempeh, Daiya brand cheese, and a package of Tofurky or Field Roast veggie sausages.

The crisper drawers hold all kinds of veggies—greens, broccoli, cabbage, and peppers are regular residents—plus apples and lemons. And, the door of the refrigerator holds many of my favorite condiments: Vegenaise brand vegan mayo, spicy mustard, ketchup, walnut oil, miso, and tahini.

The freezer is crammed with homemade black bean burritos (I make a huge stash of them to last a month), homemade veggie burgers, frozen vegetables and all kinds of nuts which I buy in bulk. There's a little vegan ice cream in there, too!

BEYOND DIET: LIFESTYLE TO PREVENT AND CONTROL CHRONIC DISEASE

A healthy vegan diet can be a powerful way to maintain your health through the decades. It's not the whole story, though. The foods you eat are just one part of a healthy lifestyle. Needless to say, ditching tobacco is an important step toward optimal health. And so are exercise and stress management.

GET MOVING FOR YOUR BODY AND BRAIN

Finding an exercise program that you love can do wonders for your health and happiness. It doesn't have to be time consuming or strenuous. Thirty minutes of brisk walking every day and a modest program of weight training two or three times per week can be enough to reap substantial benefits.

Exercise improves insulin sensitivity and reduces inflammation.[51] In fact, brisk walking for at least three hours per week or more vigorous exercise for one and a half hours per week can lower your risk of heart disease by 30 to 40 percent.[52] Adding a flexibility component, such as yoga to your exercise program can reduce heart disease risk, too. Better flexibility is associated with suppler arteries, which can counter hypertension and heart disease.[53]

Strength training is important, also, because it prevents muscle loss as you age and may even reverse it.[54] And it's crucial for the health of your bones. Being a couch potato is one of the worst things you can do for bone health. Certain exercises will also improve your balance, reducing your risk of falling.

Finally, physical exercise is great for your brain. It's possible that being physically active increases factors in the brain that are involved in neurological repair.[55] And researchers have found that just three sessions of aerobic exercise per week actually increases brain volume in people over the age of sixty.[56] Research shows fairly consistently that people who exercise regularly are at lower risk for dementia.[57]

TAMING STRESS IS POWERFUL MEDICINE

Changes that come with the passage of time can be sources of stress and sometimes depression—reduced income, worries about health, changes in identity that come with retirement, and loss of loved ones. You've already seen that a vegan diet answers some of these concerns—those about our legacy, our health, and the continuing impact of our choices. But if we feel overwhelmed by stress or depression, it can take some time and attention to manage that.

Managing stress is powerful for prevention of disease. Stress is linked to chronic inflammation[58] and therefore can raise the risk for heart disease, hypertension, and diabetes. Stress may also raise the risk for dementia, as it's been shown to suppress production of new nerve cells in the brain.[59]

It's also not surprising that the things we know are helpful in reducing stress, such as exercise and meditation, are also linked to less inflammation.[60] And inflammation itself may promote depression.[61] It doesn't mean that you can cure clinical depression with a healthy diet, but it's certainly something that can't hurt. Be sure you are also getting adequate vitamin B_{12}, vitamin D, and the long-chain omega-3 fats DHA and EPA. Shortfalls of any of these may make depression worse.

If you suffer from depression or find yourself overwhelmed by and unable to cope with stress, seek help from your health-care provider. At the same time, take advantage of simple lifestyle choices that can ease symptoms of stress and depression:

- Make sure you get plenty of sleep.

- Exercise daily. A brisk walk can do wonders for stress management. When the weather permits, try to get outside for a walk and enjoy the restorative power of nature.
- Take advantage of your social support systems. Call or get together with friends. Check meetup.com to find local interest groups, or even start one devoted to veganism.
- Meditation and relaxation techniques appear to be powerful ways to manage stress. They are associated with improved immune function[62] (ever noticed that you are more likely to get a cold when you're extra stressed?) and the management of blood pressure.[63] Meditation techniques that foster compassion may also reduce inflammation and create healthier responses to stressful situations.[64]

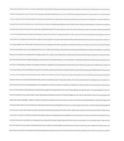

PART THREE

EATS WELL WITH OTHERS

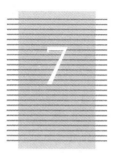

RELATIONSHIP DYNAMICS:
FAMILY AND FRIENDS AND VEGANISM

ATING IS OFTEN a social event. We "break bread" with loved ones, friends, co-workers, and with groups with which we are affiliated. A change in what you are eating will not go unnoticed. Instead of breaking bread, it may feel as if you have broken something else. In this chapter we will discuss the changes that may occur in close relationships when you become a vegan. In the next chapter, we'll consider changes in the larger social context, including going out to eat.

We hope that most of your friends are supportive of you and that your family applauds you, but that is not always the case. You may feel excited and energized by the decision to be a vegan. Sadly, many may not embrace your decision positively. If they behave like many of the families and friends we know you will meet resistance, teasing, defensiveness, and arguments as well as behavior that can range from petulance to sabotage.

Don't be alarmed; because these behaviors are so predictable, you know in advance they're not about you—and not really about them, either.

Think about the food choices we have been encouraged to make in our lives: we likely grew up conditioned by our society to view meat, dairy, and eggs as healthy food choices. Until 1992, two of the four basic food groups (adopted in the first decade of the baby boomer era in 1956) were meat and dairy.

Give yourself credit for the independent thinking, wisdom, and compassion in your decision to be a vegan. Knowing that all your previous years have led to this decision, you should feel comfortable and confident in claiming your choice now.

SITUATING YOURSELF

POSITIVE COMMUNICATION

Family counselors have a saying, "She changed but forgot to tell others she changed." In other words, issues in relationships often arise not because of the change that occurred, but due to a failure to discuss what brought about the change and what it means.

With veganism, it is a little different. To begin with, dietary changes are usually obvious. More important, changing our diet has an effect on others. If you are the kind of person who avoids arguments and will do almost anything to keep the peace, going vegan might present you with an invaluable opportunity to grow. A marvelous book, by Deborah Day Poor, *Peace at Any Price: How to Overcome the Please Disease* teaches us that we surrender our own well-being when we compulsively put others' feelings and needs before our own. We may disappoint others with our choices, but we can survive their disappointment when we hold firm with kindness and honest communication. When we learn to speak from our own truth and from our own, personal experience, we learn to tolerate with less and less discomfort the discomfort of others.

You can say, "I need you to know that I am going vegan. I am doing this for my health, the well-being of the animals, and the planet. I am asking for your support as I explore what this means for me." Explain that you are not asking people to change. Enroll them in the process. Tell them it's not because you have decided to become difficult. You can say, "I learned what happened to animals and I couldn't do it anymore." You might want to tell your family, "I'm sparing you the details about what I learned."

If sharing books is a part of your relationship, you could show them this book and summarize its argument. Sarah Taylor, who blogs at thevegannextdoor.com and is the author of *Vegan in 30 Days*, reports that she "bought copies of *Diet for a New America* for all my closest family members and friends when I first went vegan. I included a card that said, 'Please know that by sending you this book, I do not expect you to go vegan. As my sister/mother/friend/etc., I just want you to understand why I have decided to go vegan, and alleviate any concerns you may have about my health. Please read this simply as a favor to me, so I feel like you can at least understand my reasoning, and hopefully feel you can respect my choice.'"

BE PREPARED FOR AND UNDERSTAND PUSHBACK

New vegans are often surprised when what they feel is positive is treated so negatively by others. What is at the heart of this resistance? Our embrace of veganism does not happen in a vacuum. *Until a vegan enters a room, the others aren't meat eaters; they are simply eaters.* When we leave some foods off our plates, or in any other way unintentionally remind others that we are vegans, we cause them to have consciousness about what they are eating. Our choice has suddenly defined them. This reminds them that they have a choice; a choice they might never have consciously recognized before, or a choice about which they feel uncomfortable or even defensive.

Others may interpret your decision as being about them (if they aren't vegan). This prompts their emotional responses. But they also anticipate that your decision is going to have an effect on them. They fear that you are going to inconvenience them, deprive them of beloved or tasty food, or preach veganism to them.

Incompatibility does not arise from differences; it arises from whatever prompts them to stand out. No matter how much media attention veganism has garnered, be prepared for others to be totally in the dark about what it is you actually eat.

Nonvegans may associate their meals with abundance and vegan meals with scarcity and self-denial; many still think vegans eat only beans, granola, tofu, and rice. You yourself are probably still learning all the varieties of food choices that opened up when you decided to get your nourishment from plants. If this is the case, you can share your pleasure in these meals.

Nonvegans fear that being vegan is very hard. Eating delicious food is not hard. But fearing scarcity—or worse, feeling that the vegan is making food decisions about what they themselves should be eating causes many nonvegans to get upset when they are presented with a vegan meal. Nonvegans don't like to feel someone is depriving them of their right to eat what they want to eat. In Living Among Meat Eaters, Carol coined this maxim: People are perfectly happy eating vegan meals as long as they don't know that's what they are doing.

Expect defensiveness and know how to diffuse it by redirecting the discussion and not responding defensively yourself. But understand that you aren't the cause, nor are you the solution, to someone's defensiveness and anxiety. (See page 155 for more about communication.)

TRADITION. TRADITION! TRADITION?

New vegans sometimes find holidays challenging. When decades of tradition bump up against your new vegan choices, there can be tension in the weeks leading up to the big day. Rest assured, any holiday events that you enjoyed in the past will still be enjoyable now. You can serve one or more main-dish recipes from this book and be confident that you, and anyone who shares them with you, will be glad you made them.

If you are invited to someone else's home for a holiday meal, you will probably want to offer to bring a dish to share. If the host says that it's not necessary, then you might want to mention that you are a vegan and that you would be more comfortable bringing one dish that you know you will be able to eat. Even if you are the only vegan at the table, you will then be able to eat what you choose, participate fully, and leave satisfied.

Holidays are most often "eat and let eat" affairs, with vegans and meat eaters sharing a table in peace. Some vegans may feel uncomfortable about having a turkey or lamb or pig on the table. It may feel too difficult to partake with others who still eat these animals. But many vegans look at holidays more as a chance to connect with loved ones and they focus on the foods they can eat, not on what is unappealing.

If you are hosting a holiday meal in your home, you may choose to share recipes with family members or friends and ask them to bring a vegan dish. Many hosts make the main course and dessert and ask others to bring vegan sides.

In a family, preparing and sharing food represents love, nurture, and nourishment. Sometimes family members will have invested the food items themselves with emotional meaning. A mother's love, or a grandmother's or a father's, is represented in the meat dishes they always made.

Because your veganism may be seen as negating tradition, this might create disappointment or pushback. Often it is the older generation that is seen as the determiner and the carrier of the tradition. Now, instead of maintaining tradition within the home, you are seen as the one changing the tradition.

5 TIPS FOR AFFIRMING FAMILY TRADITIONS AND YOUR VEGANISM

1. **Make a *new* tradition out of the *old*.** Veganize the family's favorite recipes. You may be surprised to learn that herbs and spices impart the same familiar flavors when they are added to plant foods as they did when they were seasoning meat. But at first, don't remind people that this is what you have done.

2. **Make a *new* tradition out of the *new*.** Brainstorm with your family members about their favorite cuisine and create a meal based on that. Or have a pizza or pasta bar, with all the (vegan) makings for each person to craft his or her own dish. Or research your cultural heritage and find out what vegan foods have always been a part of it.

3. **Make up a title to a recipe that can be specific to family members or the event, such as "Giving Thanks Stuffing."** It inaugurates a tradition. Our mind is associative. It likes to put two and two together. Giving titles to recipes speaks to this associative desire. Then we simultaneously feed the person, feed the memory, and feed the mind. We prepare people for the following year, when we make the same dish.

4. **Get your family involved as sous chefs in the kitchen.** If you have always been the only one the kitchen, bring more people in there with you. Having sous chefs will demystify the process of cooking vegan. Moreover, if you are preparing an ambitious feast, it will speed the process. Starting a new tradition begins with asking people to help.

5. **Remind people that the heart of tradition is being with one another,** hearing stories, being a part of one another's lives and, in these acts, creating new memories.

YOUR FAMILY

Different types of relationships raise different issues. How you communicate with your partner about your vegan diet, for example, is likely to be different from how you talk with adult children about it.

YOUR PARTNER

If you are the primary food preparer, you may not want to prepare meat or dairy any longer. You may want your partner to embrace these exciting changes with you. And maybe that will happen. But all is not lost if it does not.

As we have said, begin with positive communication. Enlist your partner's support. But expect there may be some frustration; if responsibility for some aspect of preparing food is your role, more has changed than your diet. What will your partner eat now?

According to the reports we received in almost all (maybe really all) of those situations when partners don't agree to go vegan, the partner winds up eating way less meat and other animal foods. So that's a positive note for those who might find themselves struggling in a nonvegan family. Phyllis reported that she announced to her husband, "I wasn't going to eat or cook meat anymore because of what I'd read. He was furious—possibly because I made a radical decision on my own that would affect him. He eventually went along with the new eating regimen, but for years drank dairy milk and ate butter and eggs while I switched over to nondairy equivalents. He still puts a little butter on corn on the cob, and buys his own cheese now and then, but has made great strides, I think."

Communication every step of the way is very important, though at some point your partner may long for those days when food wasn't such a conscious decision each day. Often when people change their daily habits, especially habits associated with comfort, their partners feel as if rug has been pulled out from under them. Give your partner hugs and compliments and make an effort to say, "I love you."

You can say, "This is what I can no longer do. I can't fix hamburger/chicken/turkey any more. I'm still going to love you through my food, I'm going to love you inside out, because the food is so much better for you, and I hope you come to like it as I have. But even if you don't I still love you, and I would welcome your support in this adventure I am on." (If you don't prepare food, but usually go out, see the next chapter on getting tasty vegan food at restaurants.)

5 POSSIBLE WAYS TO INCORPORATE VEGANISM INTO AN ESTABLISHED RELATIONSHIP

1. The household will be vegan, but your significant other could choose whatever he/she wants when eating out.

2. Serve side-by-side meals; that is, foods that can be vegan and nonvegan simultaneously (two kinds of spaghetti sauce, sandwiches, etc).

3. "You can fix it." The household will not be vegan, but if your significant other wants something nonvegan, he or she will learn to prepare it: "I will fix a main course (pasta, stir fry, burritos), and you can fix the meat that could accompany that dish."

4. Your partner's kind of foods are prepared your kind of way: "I will learn how to prepare foods that make you not miss the meat." Veggie meats such as texturized vegetable protein, seitan, tofu hot dogs, or veggie burgers, could become prominent in your list (see chapter 10, "How to Veganize"). Perhaps your significant other will experiment with you, even to the point of becoming your sous chef as you develop new recipes. If you like to cook, make notations on the recipes of those that garnered the highest praise.

5. You may enjoy going your separate ways, such as a meat eater's night when your partner cooks or orders in while you go out to eat by yourself or dine with a friend

YOUR CHILDREN

Unless they were vegans before you, adult children may have strong reactions to your decision. They sometimes don't want this kind of change in their family home. They've left home and when they come back they want everything undisturbed, especially the foods they associate with growing up.

Your role is not so much to continue feeding them meat and dairy if you no longer wish to prepare it, but to ease them through these new differences so that the changes don't stand out.

Tell your children why you are becoming a vegan, and enlist their support.

If they want the traditional meals fixed in the way they used to be fixed, give them the recipes and encourage them to try them at home.

Yet you may hear: "It's not going to be the same coming home, without the family traditional meal." Or, "You don't love us." In other words, *you took care of us by feeding us, and now you are not going to feed us what you taught us to expect.* It's as if you are breaking an implied promise.

You can say, "I love you, but I can no longer prepare the foods I used to prepare." It is often difficult for young children to recognize that their parents' interests are indeed separate from their own. It is important that children, especially adult children, have the ability to recognize that one's parents have desires and needs for themselves. The adult child may actually have never examined the childish belief that their parents exist only to take care of their children's needs. Your veganism calls attention to the fact that you have the right to your own desires. You may remind your adult child why you are doing this, for your health, the animals, the planet, and tell them, "I hope you can see I am happier/healthier and I hope that you will be happy for me." It is probably good for adult children to learn to empathize with you. (It's good preparation for any future caregiving roles they may have in your life!)

OUR VEGAN LIVES

What's in Our Vegan Homes

Patti: Except for shoes and underwear, I try to buy as much as I can from stores that sell gently used clothing. Many thrift stores benefit wonderful organizations or help train people to work. In my area there are thrift stores that benefit our local Humane Society, a suicide hotline, a hospice, and an organization that provides clothing to people who need but cannot afford clothes for work or job interviews. And because cotton is one of the most heavily sprayed crops, reusing cotton clothing reduces our use of pesticides and herbicides. I love that the clothes I buy at these stores help the planet (less waste, fewer resources, fewer chemicals), people, animals, and my wardrobe!

Carol: I like to support local artisans and buy pottery serving dishes. Then when I have people over to dinner I serve the vegan dishes I have prepared in these lovely colorful and beautifully glazed pottery dishes; I see this as a way of announcing, "You are going to have an aesthetically pleasing experience at this meal!" I like to think of it as trumpets announcing the entrance of something grand, and the something grand is a plant-based meal.

In my closet you will find two pairs of vegan cowboy boots. Because I live in Dallas, it is fun to wear them to special events. This provides an opportunity to show that even cowboy boots can be vegan! I have a few favorite vegan-friendly shoes, such as Merrell's Encore Breeze and Dansko's Mary Jane shoes (which for some reason they call Valerie not Mary Jane!).

I use cloth backpacks and computer bags from Vera Bradley—colorful and convenient.

Ginny: Vegan fashion is fun! My favorite handbag, made by Big Buddha (a vegan company) is a somewhat dramatic one embellished with huge pleather (artificial leather) roses. I get comments and compliments on it everywhere I go and people are always surprised to hear that it's not leather. I also love the little fabric handbags that abound at craft fairs—almost always vegan and inexpensive.

I often buy shoes online from Zappos; it's not a vegan store, but it has a great selection of vegan shoes, and the shipping is free, which makes it easy to sample lots of different styles.

Once I have my accessories taken care of, clothes are a breeze for me since my wardrobe is mostly jeans and cotton tees. I have a few rayon dresses that will see me through any dress-up occasion. And in the winter I warm up with cozy polyester fleece.

Even though my own style is ultracasual, I love reading vegan fashion blogs. A couple of favorites are jesseanneo .blogspot.com. and totalimageconsultants.com/blog. I also read thediscerningbrute.com to stay up on vegan fashion and lifestyle ideas for my husband.

You'll also find mountains of yarn all over my house made from natural fibers, such as soy, bamboo, Tencel, and even corn, since I'm relearning to knit and crochet (haven't done either since I was a teen).

And finally, I'm a bit of a glutton for nail polish, hand cream, bubble bath and other little luxuries. It's so wonderful that cruelty-free versions of all of these products are available everywhere these days—from health food stores to Walmart. I find it helpful to shop with the phone apps Be Nice to Bunnies and Cruelty-Free to help me find products that have no animal ingredients and that haven't been tested on animals. And if something is hard to find, I turn to online stores, such as Pangea or Vegan Essentials.

YOUR PARENTS

For every year we age, so do our parents, if they are still alive. They might be shocked that we are refusing traditional foods. They may be wondering, *why aren't you eating the way you always did?* They may be confused, resistant, and downright hostile to your change in diet.

While we object to stereotypes of aging people, we have found that many octogenarians and nonagenarians like to follow the habits they are comfortable with: dinner at a certain time, a television show or not, reading the newspaper after breakfast, saunas on Saturday at one, volunteering on Mondays and Wednesdays, afternoon walks or naps. When we come to visit, we unintentionally throw all of that off. At mealtimes, we're an additional person at their table.

As vegans, we might need to decline to eat the foods our parents prefer to buy or prepare. We may be bringing new foods into their refrigerator. We might offer to cook for them. Things that seem a natural part of how *we* relate to our parents are no longer the accustomed part of how *our* parents relate to us.

Of course, as over-fifty vegans, we probably know how to be diplomatic and not push our diet upon our aging parents. But all the small changes that occur just by having a visitor in a house may result in uneasiness and anxiety for them. Looking for an explanation of these unexpected and disconcerting feelings, an obvious one rears itself—it's your veganism. A visit that we think is going well may not be going equally well for our parents. And sometimes we discover that those childlike needs for affirmation and acceptance long dormant in our adult lives spring to life in a moment of unplanned and undesired confrontation with elderly parents.

One over-fifty woman was visiting her ninety-something parents. Her father was a retired chemist whose work had helped bring about the green revolution. We'll let her son describe what happened: "Needless to say, he is not too receptive to the idea that big agriculture isn't the savior of the world that people of his generation thought it would be, and he openly disparages Mom's efforts to eat differently. At one point during the visit, he was complaining about the vegan meal that my mom had made for my grandmother and him (virtually indiscernible from the food they usually eat, mind you, thanks to my mom's creativity and resolve), and he went on an unsolicited rant about how they make concessions to Mom's dietary practices when she is there, but she won't cook meat for them when they visit. My mom pushed back a little bit against her father's bullying, and to her shock and deep dismay, her mother—always a very warm, loving, compassionate, and conflict-averse person—spoke up and said that our family's vegan diet was creating 'a rift in the family.' Mom was so crushed that she left the table and started texting my sister and me for support. She was totally bewildered."

Philosopher Alan Watts once said people eat the menu, not the meal.

The idea that a change of a diet is a betrayal of one's parents, or is even about one's parents, is an example of that. What was best for us was the love that came with the pot roast, not the pot roast itself. The love and the intention that came with the food we were fed by our parents may have enabled us to grow into mature adults. So, what should we do in such a situation? At a calmer moment, you might gently say that you are grateful to them for raising someone who is a lifelong learner. That you are thankful they raised someone who is capable of taking care of himself or herself, even if those ways differ from theirs.

And we have to honor and respect and be grateful for the care that our parents provided for us.

But we also have to recognize that for a variety of reasons, they may find it difficult to accept our vegan diet. It's that much more difficult for us to be blamed and criticized about our choice when we are trying so hard to show elderly parents our love, to be fully present to them, to cherish each moment of time we have with them.

As we said at the beginning of the chapter, this kind of behavior is predictable. You learn that no matter what loved ones say, it's not about you, and it really isn't about them, either.

DINING WITH FRIENDS, OR NOT: AVOIDING BEING UNINVITED

Meals shared with friends are an important part of socializing for many of us. Perhaps you and your spouse regularly go out to eat with another couple. Maybe a group of friends takes turns hosting dinners. You may live in a retirement community and participate in a games night—playing cards after a shared meal.

Not only do we enjoy our time with good friends, but this time with friends is actually good for us! Studies indicate the social support is a contributor to good health. It is said that the i in *illness* is also for *isolation*. And the first two letters of *wellness* remind us that partnership is good for us.

In the surveys Patti and Carol received in 2011, a notable difference appeared between vegans under age fifty and people who had become vegans after fifty. Sadly, what many over-fifty vegans reported was they were no longer being invited by friends to join them for a meal.

In 2013, Ginny invited vegans over fifty to share their experiences with her. This same heartbreaking pattern was reported. Phyllis wrote, "As for challenges, our social lives have been cut back because most of our friends are omnivores, eat the 'traditional' foods on holidays, and therefore we aren't invited to their traditional gatherings." A woman in her sixites, Carol, wrote Ginny: "This has been the most difficult thing I have ever done. I have felt alone and sad much of the time. I live in a fifty-five-plus village and most people here do not understand at all. We no longer receive invitations from friends to join them for dinners and other functions. My husband was taken by surprise and was very reticent to change. In fact, he still claims he is not vegan but has agreed to eat more and more vegan dishes with only occasional meat added. Cooking has been a huge learning curve with no support other than reading online blogs. Every social experience comes with angst and fear, but with each encounter, I am growing stronger and more confident."

None of our correspondents regretted becoming vegan. They felt their veganism was a positive addition to their lives. But they did regret the diminished social interactions they were now experiencing. Ginny's correspondent, Carol, continued, "Despite the struggles I have had, I have no doubt whatsoever that this is the right path for me and acting on what I know is right is one of the things I am most proud of. Sometimes the most difficult decisions are the most worthwhile."

BEING UNINVITED: WHY DOES IT HAPPEN?

While we don't know why their nonvegan friends ended these social get-togethers over meals, several of our correspondents speculated as to the reasons:

Phyllis wrote, "Maybe we're perceived as weird, or just having cumbersome dietary restrictions, so best to just leave us off the guest list." Linda speculated that "they feel a bit guilty and self-conscious about the food on their plates when they see what's on mine, despite their protestations about the weirdness of veganism." Emily reported how frustrating it is "to hear that my friends are struggling to figure out 'what to feed me' when I am invited for dinner, as though figuring out a plant-based menu is so difficult. I also have to work hard to assert myself about what restaurants we will go to if we eat out—I sometimes feel as if others think I am ruining their fun by insisting we go somewhere that has options for me (No barbecue, please!)."

Only one person, Linda, received an explanation for the uninviting: "Some of my friends actually told me that choosing veganism means I'm a different person than they thought I was."

We can imagine several possible motivations for friends no longer inviting you to social events that involve food:

- They don't think they can prepare a meal for you.
- They think they could, but it would be a lot of work.
- They think they could, and they don't mind the work, but they fear the reactions of their spouse or the other friends who would be there.
- They don't want to change where they go when they dine out and think vegans can't get a meal where they want to eat.
- They worry you will be difficult and call attention to the differences in food choices. Or they will simply feel awkward when they look at your plate and see that your plate is not laden the ways theirs is.
- They worry their spouse or other friends will be difficult and call attention to the differences in food choices.

5 WAYS TO AVOID BEING UNINVITED

Once you understand why friends may stop inviting you for dinner, it's a little easier to get proactive and to prevent that from happening. Here are five ways to keep yourself on the guest list.

1. When you tell friends you are going to or have become a vegan, emphasize that you still value your friendships and your social time together. "I value our friendship so much, I really want to maintain our friendship and I want you to know this isn't going to be an issue when we eat together. Please continue to invite me to dinners. They don't need to be vegan meals. I am happy to contribute a dish to any meal you plan." You could put your vegan diet in perspective by comparing it to other forms of diets (gluten-free, salt-free, diabetic, etc.).

2. Tell them you have learned from this book that invitations to dinner and relationships with friends often change. That you'd like to make sure this doesn't happen. Keep the focus on companionship and company. You could say, "I've been reading this book about people over fifty going vegan, and one of the things people talked about was that they didn't get invited to their friends' houses. My friendship with you is important; I don't want that to happen with us. There is no need for you to feel uncomfortable about my decision. I can take care of myself and I don't mind you continuing to serve whatever you would before. And I can bring some other food we can all enjoy."

3. Be proactive and invite people to your house and serve them food that they could probably imagine themselves preparing, things that aren't foreign to them; for instance, a platter of spaghetti, sautéed veggies, and toasted pine nuts. Help them envision that they could do this in their house so that they will think to themselves, "I could make this and have a vegan over to my house for dinner."

4. Understand that dinnertime with friends is probably not the most conducive time for raving about being a vegan. Be prepared to experience some (surprising) feelings of alienation and maybe sadness as you watch your friends continue to eat what you no longer do.

5. Develop the skill to order vegan at any restaurant. (For ordering at restaurants, see the next chapter.)

Or you might want to plan a get together where food is not the focus of your socializing. A night of board games or bowling or watching a film together; an afternoon walk; a museum visit or guided tour in a nearby city are all ways to spend time with friends without food at the center of the conversations.

As with any worthwhile life change, time is your friend. Be consistent with your message of kindness. Express your affection to your friends as often and as sincerely as possible. And keep kindness to yourself in the equation, too. When, over time, others see you looking happy and well, they will likely stop focusing on what you used to do and start accepting you as you are today.

WIDENING YOUR CONNECTIONS: MAKE NEW FRIENDS AND NOURISH THE OLD

Loneliness is sometimes a part of life, but it need not be a side effect of veganism. Our old friends are priceless, and it may take time and patience for their anxieties about your veganism to be relieved. But veganism is also an avenue to make new friends. There are other vegans out there, some as new to veganism as you, some with decades of experience. Many of them would love to know you, and there are ways to find them today.

- Many vegans over age fifty are surprised to find how easy it is to meet new people at vegan potluck events (see page 169), vegan restaurant outings, or vegan cooking classes or demos (see page 171). Striking up a conversation at a natural food store or a vegan friendly café is another way to meet vegans. Don't be afraid to mention that you are a new vegan. Most vegans who hear that will lavish praise, offer help and advice, and generally make you happy that you shared your exciting news. Patti has a good friend, Lois Arrow, who is approaching age ninety, whom she met at a vegan potluck dinner. Both vegans, they exchange recipes, enjoy one another's company, and share a lunch out once a month.

■ Start a monthly luncheon or dinner get-together within your community, not just with vegans and vegetarians, but with your friends. Take turns; share recipes. Stacy reported that she lives in a fifty-five-plus community "and they even have a vegetarian 'lunch bunch,' which surprised me. I think one thing about being this age is that many people do have health problems, so are used to the idea of special diets for health (even if the idea of doing it themselves appalls them)."

■ Use your computer to reach out to others beyond your immediate community. Connect with other vegans by subscribing to and participating in vegan food and lifestyle blogs or participating in discussion groups. If you love to read, join goodreads.com and explore some of the discussion groups there. You'll find groups devoted to chatting about vegan cookbooks, vegetable gardening, the vegan lifestyle, and nutrition. Connect with people, read blogs, comment on blogs, e-mail your favorite vegan blogger/cookbook author/ writer. You will feel less alone, more connected, and may even find others who comment on those sites with whom you become e-mail buddies.

■ Attend a vegfest. These day- or weekend-long events are a fast-growing trend. They are hosted by local groups in cities around the world. Many vegfest attendees are not vegan or vegetarian—just veg-curious—so invite a few friends for a fun weekend getaway with great vegan food and speakers. Every summer, the North American Vegetarian Society hosts a five-day-long "Summerfest." Patti has seen people in their sixties and seventies, who had met on a website forum or had been e-mail buddies, finally meeting each other in person at Summerfest.

- If you live in a retirement community, contact your local vegetarian society and find out whether it would be willing to host a presentation or cooking demo on veganism.
- If you are single and interested in dating, check to see whether your community has a vegan single's group.
- When you are over fifty and dating, you can choose whether to meet your date at a vegan-friendly place. If you are meeting someone you know is not a vegan, you may not have to mention your veganism at all. Just let your actions (ordering food) speak louder than your words.

COMMUNICATION: AN EXPERT ON EVERYTHING?

As the only or the newest vegan in your social circle, you may suddenly discover you are expected to be an expert on everything. People may expect you to know everything about anthropology, nutrition, evolution, plants, predators, human physiology, sociology, biology, history, Hitler (he wasn't a vegetarian, by the way), and countless other topics. You don't have to have answers to all the questions you will be peppered with. You only have to be an expert on kindness: treat your questioners kindly. Bruce, who became a vegan when he was fifty, reported, "With friends I try not to be judgmental, and answer questions about things like sources of protein when they come up in conversation. I try to show that I have a tasty, varied, and nutritious diet without feeling deprived. I also try to remember that it wasn't long ago that it would seem to me odd and extreme to be vegan."

In fact, if you don't want to, you really don't have to answer *any* of their questions. Some questions that *sound* like sincere interest in your dietary choice may actually be attempts to erect barriers or dismiss veganism. "If humans aren't meant to eat meat, why do we have canine teeth?" Or, "What about the feelings of plants?"

These questions and others are easily answered, and you'll find plenty of information to help you do so through vegan organizations, books, and websites. But do your questioners really want those answers? Or are they just trying to keep the focus elsewhere—away from the vegan issues that cause them discomfort?

In *Living Among Meat Eaters*, Carol suggests that two kinds of people exist in the world: those who want answers to their questions and those who don't. More important than knowing the answers to their questions is having the skill to tell the difference between these people. Carol advises knowing how to stop a conversation when these conversations appear to arise from anxiety, defensiveness, or hostility.

She writes, "We've all heard the saying, 'The map is not the territory.' The problem with conversations is they keep meat eaters looking at their map. Even worse, conversations often keep us looking at their map! And their map doesn't include our territory. This is why we need to stop the conversations. . . . Moreover, the questions meat eaters ask may not be the questions meat eaters need answered. Often, the content of the conversation itself is the least important aspect of a conversation. You need to learn how to identify the question behind the question."

You should assume that for the meat eater, conversations with you function to distort and block your perspective as much as they function to convey information. This perspective accounts for our basic rules for talking with nonvegans.

5 TIPS FOR TALKING WITH NONVEGANS

1. **Don't discuss veganism with people while they are eating meat and dairy foods.** It's very likely to make them feel defensive. Just tell them that you are happy to talk about your veganism, but prefer to save the discussion for after dinner.

2. **Less is more.** Not answering may be more important than answering a question. It's a different way of holding your ground. Let people know that their questions are common ones that have been answered many times—and then point them to the Internet for answers.

3. **One-liners can do a lot of work for you.**

Them: Being a vegetarian must be hard.

You: It was harder for me to live with the awareness of what I was doing eating meat and dairy and eggs.

Them: It's not practical.

You (*shrugging your shoulders casually, in a light, dismissive manner to the concern*): It is.

4. If you are going to have a conversation with a person, the first statement you make should indicate some sort of agreement with the person: "Yes, that's an interesting point." Then you might say "Many people don't know that . . ." This allows you to provide information in a way that is not confrontational or condescending. For example, "Many people don't know that animals on farms suffer greatly. I choose not to contribute to that."

5. As vegans with friends over fifty, we need to anticipate that some of our friends may be diagnosed with diseases. We need to learn how to hold our tongues or be very diplomatic. You don't want to sound as if you are blaming the victim. Being kind means expressing loving kindness, expressing care. Share your care with your friends and let them share their fears. Don't jump in with a solution. Offer something positive and helpful instead: "I'm sorry to hear of your diagnosis. Can I prepare some meals for you? Do you need any help in the kitchen?" Or if the conversation turns toward veganism in a way that isn't blaming or hectoring, you could offer, "If you need any help with shopping, recipes, or help preparing vegan food, I've been doing this for quite a while and I'm happy to help you."

If your questioner is over fifty, offer to lend the person this book with an invitation to read it and then get together to talk with you. The Irish poet Yeats observed that the most important arguments are with ourselves. This is true for nonvegans, too. We have to know how to get out of the way of nonvegans' inner processes and allow them the opportunity for inner reflection. Remember, people are perfectly happy eating vegan food as long as they don't know this is what they are doing.

VEGANS OVER 50 TELL THEIR STORIES

"I Was Ready" | Sandy Weiland

Sandy's story: Before she went vegan, Sandy Weiland had a hierarchy of which animals she would eat. She distinguished her choices by the intelligence of the animals. She explains, "I was eating basically just chicken and turkey because I thought they were 'dumb animals.' It sounds terrible. But I didn't think they had much intelligence. I didn't eat pork because I knew that pigs were very, very intelligent. They were smarter than dogs. I could not consciously eat pork for that reason."

She's embarrassed to admit this now, but for twenty or so years she continued eating in this way. "I was visiting my brother-in-law in Oregon who raises a small number of chickens for eggs and as pets. One chicken would run up to greet him every day when he came home from work, just like a dog." She realized that chickens have their personalities and saw how they treat their young. But she continued to eat "free-range," "happy" chickens and turkeys. "I was ignoring my conscience."

One day when she was fifty-four she was heading home from the grocery store and heard part of an interview with Carol on NPR news. Carol was asked, "What's the harm in drinking milk and eating cheese? That's not killing them."

Sandy listened as Carol replied, "Have you ever been to a dairy farm? The cows, when they are separated from their young, grieve for them and they search for them. If you could hear the mother cow wailing and howling for her calf and the calf crying for his mother, you would know that they mourn for each other. Male calves live miserable short lives in the dark to become veal."

Sandy had never thought of the cows being maternal and this idea "struck me to my core and so saddened me . . . I actually felt like I could hear the cows crying. It is hard to explain. That was the tipping point to decide I will not eat this anymore. It was enough for me to realize that I couldn't consciously drink the milk or eat the cheese."

The interview on NPR touched Sandy so deeply that she stopped eating all animal products that day: "I was an omnivore one day and a vegan the next."

Yet, even as she fully embraced being a vegan, Sandy found herself missing foods that she had been preparing for years. How was she going to make her traditional recipes without using meat or dairy?

Sandy began what would be a long learning curve. She experimented with making her own seitan and came up with her own meat substitute to be able to continue to use all of her favorite recipes that called for meat.

Her husband asked her, "If you are vegan, why do you want to use a meatlike substitute?" She replied, "Bill, all these years I've been cooking a certain way. I need to be able to use my traditional recipes."

Sandy also began to veganize dairy dishes. Now, she is giving out her veganized recipes "like you wouldn't believe." One of her most popular is broccoli fettuccine Alfredo, which uses homemade cashew cream. People ask over and over again for the recipe. Other friends say, " I wish you would cook for me."

When she became a vegan, her middle daughter said to her, "Mom, you are a freak. Not too many people would just give everything up at once." And Sandy said, "I was ready."

Now her middle and eldest daughters (age twenty-eight and thirty-one) have embraced a vegan diet, too.

Sandy reiterated that she did it for the animals. "I feel so good that I do not have to eat something dead to live!" She also reported, "The healthy by-product of being vegan has been outstanding. I am the healthiest I have ever been in my life. I started out not eating meat and dairy for the animals and ended up with so much more!"

As Sandy talked with us about her veganism, vegan lasagna was cooking in the oven.

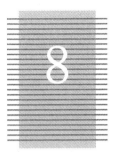

VEGAN IN THE WORLD

WHEN WE ARE home with our recipes and books, going vegan may seem like the easiest thing on earth. When we step outside into the larger world, we may encounter challenges that make us wonder whether we are doing the right thing. We *are* doing the right thing. Every roadblock we encounter as a new vegan has been overcome by vegans before us.

In this chapter, we are happy to share what we and countless other vegans have learned. Our aim is to help you triumph over any obstacles blocking your way. Of course, we cannot anticipate every possible situation. But over the years, and in survey results we have seen, the same kinds of questions come up again and again: How will I be able to go out to eat with friends? What do I do about family gatherings where vegan food is unheard of? What about birthday parties? What about feeling like I'm the only vegan in my town? People report that these challenges were daunting. Yet everyone we heard from also told us that they had no regrets about their decision to go vegan. In just about every instance, patience, time, and a commitment to kindness all help to make it easy being vegan in the world.

SOCIAL CHALLENGES

BIRTHDAY PARTIES

You will certainly not have to give up singing and celebrating birthdays when you are a vegan. Birthday cakes are usually made with eggs and butter, and as a vegan you won't be sharing the traditional cake. But birthday parties are not as challenging as new vegans fear they might be. Have you ever been at a party where a guest says, "No thank you," when the cake is offered? Maybe the person wishes to avoid gluten or sugar. As a vegan, you always have the option to say simply, "No, thank you." People will be so busy eating their own slice of cake, nobody will notice if you don't take one yourself.

And if you don't like that option, and if you are in charge of the party, then ensuring the cake is vegan is fairly simple. You can make your own (the Hummingbird cake on page 321, the Banana Cake on page 325, and the Texas Sheet Cake on page 323 make wonderful birthday cakes; or do an Internet search for "vegan birthday cake"). If you live near a Whole Foods Market or have a vegan bakery in your neighborhood, you can order one with a few days' notice. (You may be surprised to learn you indeed do have a vegan bakery nearby. Do an Internet search and find out.)

If you are a guest, you might want to bring a small cake that can be served in addition to whatever the host is serving. Or, to be different, you may want to bring vegan cupcakes instead. Also, if you are not traveling far, you can bring a vegan frozen dessert to serve with the cake. These have come a long way in the last few decades, including creamy, flavorful options made from coconut, soy, or rice milk. Any natural foods store and many grocery stores have a selection of vegan frozen desserts, including fruit-based sorbets.

Alternatively, you can bring a fruit plate that can be served along-side the cake. Many people will appreciate this option, even if they are not vegan. Patti once served a gorgeous fruit plate to her husband on his birthday, replete with candles in the melon and melted vegan chocolate over the strawberries. You could also prepare the Marzipan and Strawberries in Chocolate (see page 320).

Vegans like to celebrate as much as anyone else, and we certainly don't skip parties. A little preparation can make things easier if you are the lone vegan at the celebration. You might eat a filling meal before going to a party. Or ask if you can bring something to share. A bowl of nuts, a dip and crudités, or a platter of prepared fruit are all easy and often gratefully accepted. While it's disappointing when we can't partake of the food at a celebration, we can still focus on what we *can* partake of—the people, the happy occasion, the affection and the community. As you become more comfortable and confident in your veganism, you may find that future parties become, well, a piece of cake!

A NOTE ON CHOCOLATE

MOST, BUT NOT ALL, dark chocolate is vegan. Check the ingredients for whey, milk solids, milk, or other dairy products that are sometimes added to dark chocolate. Many vegans share with human rights activists concern about how cocoa beans used to make chocolate often come from countries where child labor (and even what some have characterized as slave labor) has been identified. The Food Empowerment Project at FoodIsPower.org provides an approved chocolate list; it even has a free app for smart phones so you can look at the list while you are shopping.

INVITATIONS TO SOMEONE'S HOUSE WHEN YOU ARE NOT CLOSE FRIENDS

Your boss invites you and your partner to dinner in her home. She doesn't know you are vegans. What to do? What to say?

Kindness, gratitude, and honesty are the key to successful relationships, even when a situation seems fraught with the potential for disaster. You might reply, "Thank you so much for asking us. That's a lovely invitation. I do need to mention that we are vegans, and that shouldn't be a problem. We would love to bring a vegan dish to share. Would that be okay?" And once you are discussing the menu, you might add, "If any cheese could be served on the side instead of mixed in, that would be wonderful." Once it is known that a vegan guest is coming, there will likely be other foods prepared that vegans can eat. Even if that's not the case, if you bring a dish of your own, you can be sure that you will have at least one dish to enjoy.

If your host is not familiar with what *vegan* means, you might mention that you are a strict vegetarian and do not eat meat, dairy or eggs. If this is a deal breaker, you might invite the boss and her partner to your house instead, to offer them a vegan meal and demonstrate that vegan food is not all that challenging. If you are the first vegan your boss knows, you can make an outstanding first impression with your generosity, honesty, gratitude, and kindness.

CIVIC OR OTHER SOCIAL BUFFETS

Sometimes, when a buffet is offered at an event, there may be no way to determine if anything at all is vegan. You can ask the servers, but they may not know. You can try to ask the kitchen staff, but even they may not know, as food is often brought in from outside catering companies. If you find yourself at a buffet with no vegan options, enjoy a cup of tea or coffee. Patti often keeps some dried fruit in her bag, or eats a big meal before attending meetings where food might be on offer. If people say, "Aren't you eating?" you can tell them that you have already eaten or that you are saving your appetite for a big meal later in the day.

When you bring your vegan dish to a neighborhood, community, or religious organization buffet, be sure to take your own portion first. When people don't know that the dish is vegan, they are likely to gobble it up before you have time to go back for seconds. All kinds of salads, macaroni and cheese, and any other veganized food will look familiar and fit right in at the buffet. Nobody will know it's vegan except you. If anyone asks you for the recipe, you can offer to send it and leave it at that. Proselytizing is not necessary, and might be counterproductive. It's usually best to let the delicious food speak for itself. Of course, if somebody asks you about your vegan diet, talk about it as you deem appropriate.

FUNERALS AND WAKES

As people over fifty, we are going to be losing our older relatives and friends if we haven't already. Grieving involves food at wakes, memorials, and houses in mourning. Loving friends and relatives often arrive with food in hand to ease the stress on the bereaved. If someone asks, "How can I help you? Can I come visit?," it is fine to say, "Yes, and can you bring something vegan?" Ask for what you need, especially when you are vulnerable and grieving.

When you bring food, it is always appropriate to bring vegan food.

A fruit plate might be very welcome. Or be inventive and create a vegan deli tray, arranging some of these ingredients on a platter:

- black olives
- sun-dried tomatoes
- marinated artichokes
- grilled asparagus spears
- pimiento-stuffed olives
- vegan versions of salami, ham, and/or turkey slices, rolled and held together with a toothpick
- cherry tomatoes
- pickled okra
- roasted eggplant cubes
- marinated mushrooms
- bread sticks (in a glass as a holder)
- assorted vegan crackers
- vegan bread

Sharing Veganism

Patti: I teach vegan cooking classes to show people how easy it can be to leave the animal products off the plate. I always speak also on behalf of the chickens, turkeys, pigs, cows, lambs, fish, and other animals during my class, to let people know that humans are not the only ones who benefit from abstaining from animal-based foods. Every time we eat, we have a chance to clog our arteries or clean them; to load up on health-promoting nutrients or to deplete them; to save the lives of animals or to ignore their plight. I feel a sense of urgency on behalf of our air and water, our climate and our rainforests, and I want to share the empowering message that our choices make a difference.

What saddens me is that many of the people who come to the class have recently been diagnosed with a terrible disease and are trying to change the way they eat to fight back. I want to tell everyone not to wait for a frightening diagnosis, but to live in the most health-promoting way possible, starting right now.

One of my favorite parts of the class is that I can work in some food jokes during the cooking. Here's one of my favorites: A man has celery sticking out of his ears and carrots sticking out of his nostrils. He goes into his doctor's office, and the doctor says, "I can tell just from looking at you. You're not eating right." You can watch a thirty-eight-minute video of a demo I did that was recorded at a vegan festival a few years ago, at youtu.be/AYdJO5i9jMM.

Carol: I love the kaleidoscopic opportunities I have for sharing my veganism. On some days you might find me speaking on a college campus and showing "The Sexual Politics of Meat Slide Show." Afterward, a vegan reception is provided, and each campus shows its own initiative in determining what to serve. At the

University of Georgia, a full Mexican meal was offered, with vegan ice cream from a new vendor for dessert. At New York University, vegan dim sum was served. At Stanford, a Middle Eastern feast of falafels, tabbouleh, and hummus was devoured by the more than one hundred people in the audience. Each of these occasions offer nonvegans an opportunity to enjoy delicious vegan food and talk about vegan issues.

On other days, I might be working on a book, an article, or a blog about some aspect of veganism. Those days, I share veganism through my writing. Writing involves postponed gratification, since I have to imagine my readers. Eating good vegan food while writing helps me endure those days of relative isolation!

And, finally, there are days when I share veganism by preparing elaborate vegan feasts, or introducing people to vegan places to eat in Dallas, or engage in local activism or education.

Then I will have circled back to my next trip, or my next deadline. I'll settle myself in the airplane or at my desk, and take a bite of the latest sandwich I have created. One time, flying to Portland, I found myself next to a woman who was going to the same conference I was scheduled to speak at. The first class meal was not vegan, but I had along a huge homemade barbecued seitan sandwich, and happily shared it with her.

Ginny: I love to share good vegan food with family and friends as often as I can. And when people ask, I'm happy to share information about all the reasons that a vegan diet makes sense as an optimal choice.

But most of my work and outreach focuses on a different type of sharing. As I became more immersed in the vegan community over the years, I also became aware of the need for information that would help vegans eat in ways that ensure adequate nutrient intake and optimal health. My work today focuses on showing people how to eat the best vegan diet possible so that veganism is a realistic and healthy long-term choice. I share that information through my blog, my books, and speaking engagements.

I also want to clear up misconceptions about the "safety" of vegan diets. So many people are concerned about whether plant foods can provide everything we need (they can!). I try to respond as often as possible to misinformation about veganism and unwarranted concerns about this way of eating.

And because many of my dietitian colleagues aren't familiar with vegan diets (we all have different areas of expertise, after all), I work on projects with nonprofit and professional organizations in developing vegan resources to help health professionals stay up to date on vegan nutrition.

SOCIAL OPPORTUNITIES

BOOK CLUBS

People in every state and of all ages belong to reading groups, and these are a wonderful way to discuss good books and get to know other people fairly well. Not all book groups include food, but sometimes the food served is as much of a focus as the books. Some groups share a meal and others serve only snacks. Some meet at a library or bookstore, and others meet in people's homes.

Many book clubs read a book each month and discuss it. The host might be in charge of suggesting some books for the next meeting, and then the group can vote on which to read.

Other book groups meet to discuss just a few chapters in a nonfiction book each month. This takes the pressure off by not having to read an entire book that month. In Marin County, California, a vegan book group meets at a Whole Foods Market once a month. They discuss two or three chapters from a book related to vegan living, such as *The World Peace Diet* by Will Tuttle, PhD, or *Comfortably Unaware* by

Richard A. Oppenlander, PhD. You can start a similar book group by doing what this group does: list it as an event on meetup.com.

If you belong to a book group that meets at home and serves food, you can show off your favorite vegan recipes when it is your turn to host. If you are not the next host, plan to call whoever is hosting next and ask whether some vegan options can be included. Offer to bring some if the host is flummoxed by the request.

VEGAN POTLUCKS OR SUPPER CLUBS

Before the computer age, a small classified ad in a community newspaper caught the eye of Patti's husband, Stan: "Vegan potluck supper at Community Church. All Welcome. Second Sunday every month; 6–8 pm." That two-line ad changed Patti's life.

A vegan for just a few years at the time, Patti did not cook much and did not know any other vegans except her husband. They attended the dinner, and then the next, and soon they had a circle of vegan friends. Jennifer Raymond, author of *The Peaceful Palate*, was running the ad and putting on the dinners. Her cookbook was Patti's introduction to vegan cooking, and it is still her favorite recipe book decades later. When a move to a different city took Patti and Stan too far away to attend these dinners, they started their own group where they lived. The newsletter—now an electronic one—for this local group is sent each month to more than two hundred people. And while potluck dinners are not held as frequently as they once were, many members host meet-up events, such as dinners out, trips to the movies, vegan bake sales to raise money for animal causes, a book club, and potluck picnics. Members also pay for a table at the annual Earth Day celebration and hand out literature about the power of our food choices to slow climate change. A community of people has come together, grown, and enjoyed companionship, all because of that one classified ad in 1989.

Starting a vegan supper club or potluck event is even easier now. You can post an event on craigslist.org or on meetup.com. You can invite people from work, the gym, your church, synagogue, or mosque, your neighborhood, and anywhere else. Ask each person to bring a vegan dish to share with eight others. You might suggest that they bring the recipe for their dish, too. It helps if people also bring their own serving and eating utensils and a plate. To find a suitable place, ask local churches, community halls, or yoga studios if they might be able to host a dinner once a month. They may ask for a fee, and you can ask attendees to chip in a few dollars each to help cover the cost. If it's a small gathering, you can even do it in your own home.

If there are any professionals who are vegans in your area—authors, nurses, physicians—you can invite such persons to be a guest speaker. This way, your event has an attraction for even nonvegans. They can hear a short talk by the local expert. Perhaps *you* are that expert. All the more reason to hold an event to share what you know while enjoying a vegan potluck meal.

If you don't know any local celebrity vegans, you can show a film at your first gathering. Patti's favorite films for this include *Forks Over Knives*, *The Witness* (by Tribe of Heart), *Peaceable Kingdom* (by Tribe of Heart), *Earthlings*, *Fast Food Nation*, *The Cove*, and *Blackfish*.

THE VEGAN POTLUCK IN WOOSTER, OHIO

THE VEGAN POTLUCK BEGAN about three years ago as a kind of support group for a few members of Westminster Presbyterian Church (including Dave Noble, College of Wooster class of 1963 and heart specialist and college trustee Ken Shafer, College of Wooster class of 1975) who wanted to share recipes and dining experiences.

When it started growing, the group moved it out of their homes and into the church (the college's congregation in residence) and threw the doors wide open to students.

And then it really exploded. It is not unusual for 50 students to attend the monthly event, which often includes a cooking lesson from staff members at the local food cooperative and a short lecture on sustainability issues, delivered by both students and community members.

Over bowls of lentil soup, pita and hummus, stuffed cabbage, and rich brownies, sixty-year-olds and twenty-year-olds exchange cooking and recipe ideas. Most of the students who attend aren't vegan but say they come to the potluck as a way to connect with the community. "And," adds Alissa Weinmanjj (class of '15), "to get away from Lowry [the dining hall] for an evening."

[Reprinted from the *Wooster* magazine.]

VEGAN COOKING CLASSES AND DEMOS

At vegan cooking classes or demos you will learn new ways of preparing foods and meet others who are somewhere along the vegan path as well. Some vegan restaurants or vegan groups offer cooking classes. If you notice someone who is always making incredible dishes for potlucks or other occasions, invite him or her to teach a class.

You might even decide that you want to step out into the world and learn how to be a vegan by teaching others how to cook vegan! New vegans often want to share the information they are learning. Here's your opportunity! You will simultaneously be learning, teaching, and creating a support group, thereby invigorating yourself and placing yourself into the world.

Arrange to do a food demo at a senior citizens center, a retirement home, public library, or as a social event at your church, synagogue, or mosque. Check first with your hosting facility if you plan to give out food samples, since there may be some restrictions regarding this.

HOW TO CONDUCT A FOOD DEMONSTRATION: The requirements for doing a food demo are actually quite minimal. If you are using a blender or food processor, take with you a very, very long extension cord. It helps to have a sink but it is not necessary, so always bring a bowl to fill with water as an improvised sink. You should plan to demonstrate two or three recipes.

Have a checklist of what you need to bring from home:

- a rubber spatula
- spoons for serving

- paper cups or plates if you are serving samples
- vegan crackers if you are making dips or spreads
- a sharp knife
- recipes to hand out (on the back of the page of recipes, you might want to put more resources—perhaps the name of this book?)

Before starting, Patti sends around a sign-up sheet that requests e-mail addresses for follow-up. This could be the foundation for starting a local group.

Then Patti shares some background about her own move to a vegan diet. She reassures people that even if the demonstrated food is the only vegan food they eat that day, they will have a good experience of vegan food and may be more open to it the next time they have the opportunity to try it. (Some people come just for the free food sample.)

The first thing she prepares is a green smoothie. She tells the attendees, "It's understandable you might not think you'll like it." Then she makes the smoothie, using frozen mangoes, fresh bananas, soy milk, and spinach. She chooses to use spinach because it has a mild flavor that is overpowered by the mango. It's green but it will taste like a mango smoothie. She gives everyone a 2-ounce sample and everyone always wants more!

Next she makes a roasted red pepper and chickpea spread, by processing in a food processor a can of drained and rinsed chickpeas with two roasted red peppers from a jar. She offers carrot sticks for dipping into the spread. She explains that you can use it on bread, eat it with a cracker, or smear it on a tortilla and add steamed vegetables. She usually brings carrot and celery sticks for dipping. She also makes hummus and talks about how versatile hummus is (see page 249).

Patti concludes the demo with a question-and-answer period. Many people share their own stories and recipe ideas as well.

Carol presented a demo at her local library, to which she brought large quantities of kale, collards, chard, tofu, and tempeh donated by local grocers. (If you receive food from a store, be sure to credit it.) Carol's goal was to demystify these foods. She had the participants remove the stems from the kale and collards to experience their preparation. She opened the tempeh and tofu and placed them in bowls and asked people to touch them, feel them, and crumble them if they wished. She had already prepared foods for attendees to enjoy eating and presented a slide show that answered the most frequently asked questions about vegan eating.

Both Patti and Carol hand out recipes—the ones they are demonstrating and additional recipes as well.

AT WORK

If your experience is like that of many vegans, your veganism will not go unnoticed at work. Bonding with co-workers often happens around meals.

You can practice the kinds of conversational responses we recommended in the last chapter; in fact, the questions might be more frequent in a work setting. You don't have to answer people's questions and don't have to get sucked into their agenda. Simply smile and change the subject. Take deep breaths and wait for them really to be interested. You'll know when that is, according to the reports we have heard from vegans who simply practiced their habit of bringing in good vegan foods for their lunch (and having enough share). It took a few years, but some co-workers began to talk to them with interest about how they fixed their meals. Your diet will actually open up the possibility of making connections. It just takes a lot of time and patience. One vegan keeps foolproof recipes in a stack in her office, to give to people who are curious.

THE WORLD'S FASTEST SNACKS AND MINI MEALS
- ready-to-eat cereal with almond milk, ground flaxseeds, and sliced peaches

- whole-grain toast topped with almond butter
- apple slices with peanut butter
- baked tortilla chips with mashed avocado and salsa
- baked potato topped with hummus (keep a bowl of baked potatoes in the refrigerator)
- veggie burger on whole wheat bread
- coconut yogurt topped with granola and sliced strawberries

EATING OUT

Vegan options are increasingly available at all types of restaurants. Especially if you live in a big city or a college town, the vegan choices have never been better. Visit HappyCow.net to find vegan-friendly places in any city around the world.

There may be times, however, when you end up in a restaurant that doesn't appear accommodating to vegans. This is often a problem in the business world, where it's not unusual to find yourself dining with co-workers and supervisors at a steakhouse. If you have any control over restaurant choices, you can suggest vegan-friendly ones. Otherwise, we'll show you how to find a vegan meal at almost any type of restaurant.

VEGAN-FRIENDLY RESTAURANTS

If you don't have a vegetarian restaurant in your area, look for Indian, Middle Eastern, Thai, Mexican, Italian, Japanese, Chinese, and Ethiopian cuisines. There are usually plenty of vegan options on the menu. In Thai restaurants, you may want to specify that you do not want fish sauce in anything you order; that's a common ingredient. Likewise for ghee (butter) in Indian food. And in Japanese restaurants, be sure to say that you do not want fish flakes—called bonito or katsuo-bushi—on anything you order. These look like wood shavings, but are made from fish flesh and are often used as a garnish.

If you love pizza, you can still get a great pizza by ordering all the veggies (doubled) without cheese. Some pizza places now offer non-dairy cheese as an option on their pies.

RESTAURANTS WITHOUT VEGAN ENTRÉES

If you don't have a vegan or vegan-friendly restaurant near you, you can work with what you do have. Talk to the manager of any restaurant you frequent and ask whether the chef can prepare vegan options for you. Cookbook author Ken Haedrich, winner of a Julia Child Cookbook Award, explains, "He or she should be willing and able to talk to you intelligently about the sort of food you would like. And you should get the distinct impression that the chef knows something about meatless cuisine and looks at feeding you as a creative challenge, not as a pain in the patootie. If the chef mumbles something about a baked potato and the salad bar, this is not a good sign."

At some restaurants, the best vegan options are listed under the side dishes. You could order a plate with rice, mushrooms and veggies, or a potato. It may not be the ideal vegan meal, but you won't go hungry.

Or look at the components of entrées for ingredients that can be pulled together to create a vegan meal. If the menu offers a portobello mushroom and steak sandwich, and also has a chicken risotto, chances are that the chef can create a mushroom risotto for you. (Ask that no chicken stock, cream, milk, or Parmesan cheese be added to it.) If you see salmon topped with grilled vegetables, then chances are you can get pasta tossed with grilled vegetables.

As you navigate the menu, keep in mind that many soups are prepared with chicken stock or dairy products, rice may be cooked with meat stock, or beans with lard; pasta may contain eggs, tomato sauce may be cooked with cheese or meat and then strained; meat-based stocks may be used to thin sauces, vegetables may be cooked in butter, and French fries in animal fat. You may need to ask about the specifics; don't simply assume that your server knows what *vegan* means.

ORGANIZING A CHEF CHALLENGE

When musician Eleni Vlachos moved to the Durham, North Carolina, area, she discovered that the city's vegan offerings were disappointing. Her friend and fellow local musician Shirley Hale-Koslowski—who also happened to be a chef—suggested that, instead of simply asking restaurants for more vegan dishes, she challenge local chefs to create the best vegan dish. Thus was born the Bull City Vegan Chef Challenge, which eventually inspired the Global Vegan Chef Challenge (see globalveganchefchallenge.com/background).

TO CREATE A VEGAN CHEF CHALLENGE: Brainstorm the restaurants you want to challenge, and the length of time for the challenge. You could pick ten restaurants for a monthlong vegan challenge. Vlachos recommends identifying restaurants that do not already have several vegan options.

You could select a specific meal. The Durham challenge in 2012 was a brunch challenge. Because brunch is a weekend activity, they limited the participating restaurants to six to ensure that people could visit all the restaurants in a month's time. (For very specific guidelines, check out the Sacramento Vegan Challenge website, sacveganchallenge.com/more-events/sacramento-vegan-chef-challenge/for-chefs-and-managers.)

Vlachos reports that "the challenge was a huge success for restaurants, which saw a huge increase in demand for these dishes. Some nights, over half of the meals ordered were the vegan challenge entries, and for patrons—53 percent who were not even vegetarian or vegan—who got to enjoy delicious thoughtfully prepared meals, then vote on their favorites."

EATING WHEN TRAVELING

Travel as a vegan can present some challenges, but none that can't be solved. Many tour groups can accommodate vegans fairly well. Be sure to ask *before* signing up whether there can be accommodations for a vegan on the trip. Also, if traveling in other countries, ask whether there will be a translator with the group during meal-times. And remember that food markets and even supermarkets in other countries are a great source for daily fare and even gifts to take home.

FOOD FOR FLYING

The skies used to be a lot friendlier for vegans, when we could at least order special meals on most airline flights. Cost-cutting measures have limited the options, though, especially for domestic travel.

If you're flying out of a large airport, you'll most likely have luck in finding something to take on the plane. At the very least, you'll almost always find a hummus wrap or a hummus bowl with crackers (check that the wrap breads or crackers are vegan).

Airport food courts usually offer Chinese food; you can get rice and veggies and sometimes stir-fried tofu. Vegan travelers have been thrilled to discover Cibo Express gourmet markets sprouting up at airports across the country. They offer vegan sandwiches made with veggie meats.

To save money and ensure that you won't go hungry, you may want to pack your own meal. The Transportation Security Adminis-tration (TSA) treats both hummus and peanut butter as liquids, which means you'll most likely have to pack them in a resealable plastic bag and limit them to 3 ounces. Some vegans report that they have no trouble bringing these foods along in their carry-on lug-gage, however. Patti empties an entire 8-ounce container of hummus between slices of bread and brings along baby carrots to scoop out the hummus.

If you have room, you can buy single-serving packets of peanut butter or almond butter to keep on hand. The Peanut Butter & Com-pany website (ILovePeanutButter.com) offers "Easy Squeezy" packets of peanut butter in a number of different flavors for travel. Be sure to pack some crackers and a plastic knife, too.

Here are a few other ideas for airline-friendly carry-on meals:

Hummus and pita bread: Put a scoop of hummus into a 3-ounce container (that's the limit for carry-on liquids) and freeze it the night before you leave. Then toss it into your resealable plastic bag and pack some pita pockets. Once you are through security at the airport, you may want to buy a salad so you have some vegetables to stuff into your homemade pita pocket.

Grain salads: Quinoa or couscous, tossed with chopped nuts and raw vegetables, makes a satisfying meal or snack. Pack the salad in a plastic container and bring a small container of dressing in your resealable plastic bag.

Instant cups of soup: Look for "instant" black bean or split pea soup in a cup and then ask for hot water on the plane. If the cup is too bulky to fit in your carry-on bag, empty it into a plastic bag for travel and use the hot water cup for mixing.

Veggie meat sandwich: Add slices of a vegan deli meat, such as Tofurky or Field Roast, to whole-grain bread, wrap in plastic, and freeze the whole thing.

Mixed nuts or soy nuts: Add them to a green salad purchased at the airport for a protein and energy-packed meal.

GoPicnic brand hummus and crackers meal: This vegan meal-in-a-box includes aseptically packaged hummus (no refrigeration required) multiseed crackers, mixed fruit and nuts, dry-roasted edamame, and a square of organic, dark chocolate. Find it at veganessentials.com.

NOT IN A HURRY? TAKE THE TRAIN

IF YOUR TRAVEL PLANS are leisurely ones, consider Amtrak. Many of its Bistro cars offer vegan burgers as well as hummus with crackers. You can watch the scenery roll by, check your e-mail using the train's free wireless connection, and enjoy a burger and a glass of wine. Vegan travel doesn't get much better than that!

TRANSLATING YOUR VEGAN FOOD REQUESTS

The Vegan Society, in the United Kingdom, published a useful guide called *The Vegan Passport* that translates what you do and don't eat into seventy-three different languages. Although it is now out of print (and available at exorbitant prices at online book dealers), you can order one today for $8 from the American Vegan Society (americanvegan. org, 856-694-2887). You can also use the translation feature of Google to create your own message that politely explains what you would like to eat and not eat.

If you have a smart phone, you can translate your requests and questions into any language, and just show the screen to your server.

Some trips and destinations cater to vegans. Check out VegVoyages. com for information on vegetarian and vegan tours in India, Malaysia, Thailand, Laos, Bali, and Indonesia. In northern California, try The Stanford Inn, a vegan resort in Mendocino, California. To find vegan-friendly B&Bs anywhere in the world, consult HappyCow.net/ travel.html.

GETTING BETTER ALL THE TIME

Social norms are powerful. Every time people see others doing something unfamiliar, it becomes less weird to them. For many people, we may be the first vegan they ever met. For others, we may be the fifteenth or hundredth vegan they know. Our being vegan normalizes veganism. When people see vegans everywhere, we stop seeming strange. We may seem trendy. We may seem smart. Or brave. But for sure we make being vegan more "normal" when we live our lives as happy vegans in the world.

You are taking a bold and beneficial journey that will have its cheerleaders and its detractors. As you continue on your path, you will become more and more confident and adept in meeting challenges and thriving as a vegan. We are with you every step of the way.

VEGANS OVER 50 TELL THEIR STORIES

"Compassion helped get me to the next level, veganism." | Donald Moy

Donald's story: Donald Moy attended the first meeting of the Black Vegetarian Society of Texas in 2001 and has been going ever since. A vegetarian at age twenty-one, and a vegan for the past seventeen years, Moy is retired from the United States Department of Education, where he was a civil rights investigator for thirty years. In 2001, a co-worker saw a notice in an African American weekly newspaper, announcing the formation of the Black Vegetarian Society of Texas. She knew Donald was a vegetarian and called his attention to the notice. That is how he went to the first meeting. As of 2013, he was still on the board, and was its past president.

As a civil rights investigator, Donald had to deal with several federal laws: Title IX (the educational amendment of 1972 requiring equity in athletics and educational programs), section 504 of the Rehabilitation Act of 1973 (that addressed disability issues and physical accessibility to school buildings), the Age Discrimination Act of 1975, and Title VI of the landmark 1964 Civil Rights Act (that prohibited discrimination on the bases of race, color, and national origin), which he refers to as "the grand daddy of all civil rights legislation." His work required travel throughout the South and Southwest to investigate alleged civil rights violations by schools.

Traveling as a vegan was not always easy. Many places he traveled to were small towns that didn't have vegetarian restaurants. One time in West Texas, he ate at the same Chinese restaurant every night. He began to pack his food for trips. "I'd make my brown rice; I'd take some vegetarian meat substitutes and pack them with freezer packs. I'd try to get a room that had a refrigerator and a stove top or a microwave." On arriving at his destination, he would go the grocery store and buy fresh fruit and veggies. Then he could build a meal, and eat in the room.

Donald grew up as, and still is, a Seventh-day Adventist. Seventh-day Adventists teach health reform and healthy living. His family ate meat as he was growing up, but only those considered "clean meats" according to Seventh-day Adventist beliefs. He often ate vegetarian food, especially at church functions. (About 50 percent of Adventists are vegetarian.) But he loved his mom's home cooking. He grew up in Monroe, Louisiana—"If you know anything about Louisiana, we pride ourselves on our food." Once he left home, it was much easier to become a vegetarian. Being in a community of friends who were also mostly vegetarians helped him to make the transition.

Compassion began to become more central to his thought after becoming a vegetarian. "Compassion helped get me to the next level, veganism." Specifically, he learned more about how animals are treated prior to slaughter, "not to mention the slaughter itself, which is horrible." That really tugged at his heart. "I realized I didn't want to be a part of it." The biggest impediment to becoming a vegan was that he loved cheese. "That was the last thing I wanted to give up and Blue Bell ice cream, too. But tasting some of the vegan ice cream and vegan cheeses helped me to evolve and realize, 'Okay, I can do this.' One thing I love is Amy's vegan macaroni and cheese dinner (it's comfort food). Then when I looked at the back, I realized it had 450 calories! Being a fitness fanatic, I fight hard to work off the extra calories through walking, biking, and my workout passion—tennis."

As a vegan, Donald knew about other vegetarian and vegan groups, but he never joined any of them. What drew him to the Black Vegetarian Society of Texas was the name "Black." He explained that he liked being a part of a group that was trying to reach out and have an effect in his community. "When you look at the lifestyle diseases, such as diabetes and hypertension, a lot of those issues are related to how we eat and they are affecting the black community in a higher proportion than the general population." The mission of the Black Vegetarian Society of Texas is "to educate the public, particularly the African-American community, on the benefits of a plant-based diet to promote wellness and influence the community to pursue a vegetarian lifestyle." The society's educational programs are many. It holds an annual Meat Out celebration in March, with speakers on vegetarianism and health, as well as participates in various community health and ecology fairs throughout the year, offering monthly "101" classes—an introduction to plant-based eating. This class includes information on the reasons for becoming a vegetarian, covering environmental issues, compassion, and diet-related diseases. It covers how and where to shop as a vegetarian. There are also quarterly vegan cooking classes, and in the summer, a "'shopping as a vegetarian class,' where we go on-site and take people to a vegetarian-friendly grocery store to learn how to shop healthfully on a budget."

Out of respect for those who are vegans, all the society's activities are from a vegan perspective. But, importantly, it works with people wherever they are. Many people are in transition, eating chicken or fish. "We try to encourage them wherever they are. We want anyone to join as long as they have the goal in mind of healthier living."

Donald gained some additional inspiration from his mom. She went vegan after a health scare. He especially loves her vegan macaroni and cheese (see page 302 for her recipe). He enthusiastically echoed this book's title: "As you say, it's never too late to gain benefits from a vegan diet."

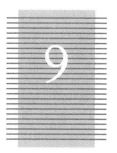

VEGANISM AND CAREGIVING

FOR VEGANS, ONE of our acts of giving care is to refuse to support a system that causes the suffering and death of animals. But, as vegans over age fifty, we may discover that another kind of caregiving has become an intimate part of our lives.

In this chapter, we are focused on a very specific form of caregiving. This kind of caregiving is: *attention that is helpful to another because of that person's physical, mental, or emotional needs.*

Someone—a parent, another relative, a close friend—may require physical, mental, or emotional support. This need for help may be temporary, creating a crisis—for instance, a broken hip, pneumonia— and then the need disappears, the crisis passes, and life returns to "normal." This is *crisis caregiving.*

Sometimes the need for assistance is coexistent with the person, and will always be there as long as the person is alive. Life takes on a new normal, the norm of ongoing care provision. This is *chronic caregiving.*

For individuals who chose to have children, they have to be Janus-faced in their caregiving: concerned both about their children and also about their aging parents or other relatives. Individuals who chose not to have children discover a different double-bind: because they do not have children, they are the ones expected to drop everything to provide care—either crisis or chronic—to an elderly relative. No matter how much you love the person you are caring for, a health crisis can be incredibly taxing and unsettling to all concerned.

Vegans may have already honed their skills at caregiving, and yet discover limits to their caregiving ability that shake their sense of self. Unlike nonvegan caregivers, vegans may discover that there are many ways in which their veganism impacts caregiving. Your being vegan may be something that enhances this experience, complicates it, and/ or may enable you to bear the burden of some of the emotional conflicts and physical exhaustion that occur during times of crisis.

We believe it is important for there to be *a theory and practice of vegan caregiving*. Even if you aren't a caregiver at this time (or a care receiver— we will get to that), you might want to review the ideas in this chapter, as it may be helpful to have some familiarity with these practical suggestions when and if a crisis occurs.

GUIDELINES FOR VEGAN CAREGIVERS

No matter what circumstances have created the need for you to respond as a caregiver to another, here are four guidelines for vegan caregivers:

1. Lower your expectations.
2. Raise your self-care.
3. Protect the boundaries you can.
4. Enjoy healthy vegan meals.

The first three represent advice Carol received when she was a full-time caregiver. But we have added the last—"enjoy healthy vegan meals"—because we see this as essential both physically and emotionally. Vegan meals can nurture you as you nurture another.

What specifically do these guidelines mean? Some of their applications will be found throughout the chapter, but in general:

Lower your expectations because, while you are caregiving, you will not accomplish everything you hope or expect to accomplish. Don't start caregiving with agendas regarding your own work—you probably won't get to them. Don't set yourself up for disappointment. As a vegan, you will also have to lower your expectations that others will remember your specific dietary needs.

Increase your self-care because, as we will discuss shortly, caregiving is very stressful. Get rest, eat well; grab small moments of self-care: five minutes of deep breathing or stretching, resting, or getting outside. Even the very quotidian act of brushing and flossing your teeth can become symbolic of self-care.

Protect boundaries: Just because you are caring for someone does not mean that you are available to care for their friends, your friends, or anyone else at the same time. It is amazing how many people want a caregiver's spare moments. You have to cultivate the art of saying no to other demands. Nor do you have to be privy to everything in the life of your care receiver. It's okay to say "TMI" ("too much information") when your care receiver is sharing inappropriate or overly personal information.

Enjoy healthy vegan meals: You do not have to go along with what everyone else is eating or wishes you to eat. Veganism is a boundary you can protect. Caregiving is precisely when you need to feel that there are some things you have control over, even as you lower your expectations. Now is not the time to subsist on chocolate. During the stress of caregiving, your meals can nourish you on many levels.

THE STRESS OF BEING A VEGAN CAREGIVER

When we are called to be a caregiver for someone we love, we want to bring a wide-open heart.

With crisis caregiving, once the crisis of the broken hip or the pneumonia or dehydration that led to hospitalization is taken care of, we can return to our own life. The wide-open heart still feels wide and open, and we know we did the right thing.

Caregiving is filled with many, many moments of grace and deep connection, and is often motivated by love and empathy. But with a situation of chronic caregiving (prompted by dementia, debility, heart disease, frailty, or many other chronic health issues), caregiving can become a costly experience, not just in terms of money, but also in terms of emotional and physical well-being. You still have a wide-open heart, but it may feel like a black hole has opened within it. You might have to move, change jobs, and accept a lower pay to perform caregiving duties. Or you may give up your job and your house to go live with and take care of a relative.

Chronic caregiving may have crisis moments—a mother with Alzheimer's breaks her hip or develops a urinary tract infection. When the crisis is solved, one returns to the norm of chronic caregiving.

Whatever the situation of caregiving, your wide-open heart knows that caregiving contains the universe. It is one person pushing another's wheelchair, or helping someone shower, or sitting next to her as she eats, and guiding the fork or the spoon. When you gather all the singular acts of caregiving together you have a universe of feeling, of kindness, of struggle, of patience, contained within it.

The vegan caregivers bring another universe within as well, that of the awareness of why they get their nourishment from plants. Sometimes, just because of the exhaustion and demands of caregiving, those two worlds, though motivated by that same wide-open heart, collide.

CAREGIVING IS PHYSICALLY EXHAUSTING

Caregiving can be very, very hard.

When you are tired, you are more vulnerable. At times, you may feel like crying, and it's okay to cry. Some scientists now believe that crying helps the body release chemicals that build up during times of elevated stress. Carol would go to her bedroom and cry for fifteen minutes and then return to her caregiving tasks, released, and ready to be attentive to another again.

At times, many people don't acknowledge the kinds of stresses caregivers are under. It is right for the focus to be on the care receiver, but as Nancy L. Mace and Peter V. Rabins warn in *The 36-Hour Day*, caregivers often become "the second patient." This is one of the reasons it is so important to lower expectations, raise self-care, protect the boundaries you can, and enjoy healthy vegan meals.

COOKING FOR A MEAT EATER

This is a difficult topic: What does a vegan caregiver do when preparing food for a nonvegan?

If your care receiver has always been a meat eater, and even though the vegan caregiver may be acutely aware that a vegan diet could be helpful for the care receiver, this is not an opportune time to enforce or even suggest a change in diets.

Many reasons exist for this recommendation:

First, as one's physical incapacities limit one's abilities, food may become a form of support or entertainment. What is desired is the food one knows and loves, the comfort food of one's childhood. If this is true for us as vegans during times of stress, it is equally true for our care receivers.

Second, food is often symbolic of control. Many people who need relatives to come and care for them (in crisis or chronic situations) feel a loss of control simply because an additional person is there in the household. When, on top of this, the care-providing interloper takes over their kitchen, preparing foods that are not customary to their household, well, sparks can fly.

Third, foods central to our own diet may physically affect our care receiver. For someone with loose bowels, too much fruit—or certain kinds of fruit—are not helpful. For someone unaccustomed to digesting beans, the introduction of beans to a meal may cause discomfort.

Many people, especially during chronic illness, are not willing to be experimented upon. Even changing the way one cooks butternut squash can be problematic. (Believe us on this one!) Additionally, many care receivers are certain they need particular foods to be healthy or to recover health, and these foods are often not the foods a vegan would advocate.

Sometimes, the most surprisingly innocuous (to you) foods or seasonings may cause your care receiver not to eat what you have prepared. Paprika? Even if the care receiver used to cook with that herself, times truly have changed. Paprika has become an exotic food. Pepper in the mushroom soup? Better not chance it. The question is not what your taste buds like, but what theirs do. This is especially true when someone has dementia and is not eating much food—every bite the person takes is an important one.

This is not the time to fix red cabbage and apples if what the care receiver is used to is boiled cabbage.

Rejected foods (which you thought of as innocent innovations) can make you feel tired or depressed. On top of that, you still need to prepare something that will be eaten.

In the best of times, one's veganism may have been a source of contention—no matter that you are over fifty. During caregiving, which may not be the best of times (!), you may be asked to do something you haven't done in years and that sunders your heart or that you find ethically challenging, such as serve hamburgers, scrambled eggs, or some other nonvegan food for someone you love.

This conflict may be one of the most difficult you will experience as a vegan.

Some of the things your care receiver loves to eat can be accommodated to a vegan diet with surreptitious changes—soups made with a vegetable base instead of chicken stock, breads (unless there is an absolute favorite), salads. You can also try a variety of vegetable-based main courses without calling attention to the fact that they are vegan.

But in the end, you may find that you are scrambling eggs for your loved one, making grilled cheese sandwiches, or even picking up a requested fast food. It is painful and yet you do it.

Lower Your Expectations

Remember the advice to lower your expectations? This is one of those times. Lower your expectations that your vegan diet can be anything more than your vegan diet.

The care receiver needs to have calories. The vegan caregiver knows the most important thing is for the care receiver to eat *something*. We may recognize that this *something* was *someone* and yet we still serve a nonvegan meal. Our wide-open heart is torn in two.

Yet as a vegan caregiver, with every personal food choice, you are offered a reminder that your perspective includes all living beings. You might not be able to do much, apart from caregiving, but by following a vegan diet, you are doing something, bearing witness.

For each day that you are a caregiver, your veganism may have to be sufficient. You still make a difference for yourself and for the other animals you personally refuse to consume.

And if you are eating a balanced vegan diet (yes, we know that sometimes feels an impossibility at this time), you are raising your self-care. In the midst of caregiving, veganism becomes a practice that can help you with stress, helping to replenish you every day.

THE EMOTIONAL CHALLENGES OF CAREGIVING

Addressing the meat-eating wishes of your care receiver is just the most obvious illustration of the emotional challenges of being a vegan caregiver.

Caregiving can be filled with ambivalence and ambiguity. It can challenge your sense of self. The haunting question that often recurs is, *What does your humanity ask of you?*

THE DISAPPEARANCE OF SELF

Sometimes, in giving yourself to caregiving, you feel as if you have disappeared. The self is obscured. You exercise purposeful control so as to give yourself to caregiving. You put yourself aside. At times, you may be raging inside, angry at someone, upset about what is happening, hurt, frustrated, and overwhelmed, and yet you summon yourself to be loving, attentive, caring.

Is this dissemblance? No, this is caregiving. Sometimes, you have to disconnect from the feeling part of you, so you can do the job without despair.

On days when you have lost sight of the grace inherent to caregiving, your vegan diet may perform the miracle of instilling grace into your day. When you are feeling isolated by your caregiving duties, veganism is a reminder of your relationship with the rest of the created order. By maintaining a vegan diet, your care is not just for one person (though that is the focus at the moment), but your care extends around the world.

After a day of being focused on very small, but important, details of caregiving, your vegan meals can give you a feeling of connection to the larger world. No matter how depleted of self you feel, at dinner you are reminded, "This is something I can affirm. I am so happy I am vegan."

Just when you need it to, at each meal, veganism reminds you of the self that you are.

DINNERTIME IN THE MIDST OF CAREGIVING

It does not matter what age we are; we generally feel good being acknowledged by our parents or older relatives or friends, for being a part of their lives.

But it may be difficult for care receivers to acknowledge what is being done for them—they don't want to believe they need help, or at least not as much as their caregiver is providing.

When multiple relatives converge to help, the differences among them are supposed to be irrelevant, and in the best-case scenarios, they mostly are. But, if in general your vegan food was only tolerated, the tensions that accompany caregiving may result in your veganism becoming a source of stress.

LOWER YOUR EXPECTATIONS THAT OTHERS WILL POSITIVELY ACKNOWLEDGE YOUR VEGANISM

If other family members are there, you will bump up against them; like you, they are probably tired. You may discover a wonderfully nurturing environment in which the one cooking for the family remembers your veganism and makes sure all meals include you. But you also need to expect that your veganism may be a satisfying target that deflects anxiety about the person who is receiving care.

This is probably not the best time for lectures from you on the benefits of veganism. Nor do you need to discuss, defend, or explain your choice. No matter how persistent another person may be, reserve your energy for caregiving and change the subject.

In other words, raise your self-care.

It is enough, for just now, that your veganism matters to you. It does not need to matter to anyone else.

Let this mantra run through your head when someone is critical or mocking of your veganism: "I'm not going to let him/her/them make me feel bad. I'm not going to let me feel bad. I don't have to feel bad because this has to do with them, not me." Then you are successfully protecting your boundaries, as well.

CHRONIC CAREGIVING AND MAINTAINING YOUR VEGANISM

With chronic caregiving (when the person is not going to get better), the caregiver goes from thinking, "This interrupts my life" to "This is my life," and cannot trace when exactly that happened. With chronic caregiving, every day is the same and every day is completely different.

Even though you know you don't want to think this, you may have already thought, *How do I forgive a care receiver for changing my life?*

And then suddenly—it's as though you have never *not* been in the midst of it—in the midst of soiled diapers, transferring from wheelchair to bed, helping someone take one slow painful step after another—there is no past, no future, just the fact that someone's body needs your help. "I" disappears. The helper—tenderer—caregiver—is there. There is no "I" to protest, to judge.

This is really the moment for upping your self-care. Step outside for five minutes. Do floss your teeth. Make sure you have healthy vegan food.

Increasing how well you take care of yourself will make you more effective. If you need to, make it like an appointment with yourself. Map out your time. There is a continuum of behavior, with self-sacrificial behavior/self-denial at one end and narcissism at the other end. The middle between these two ends is where you would have a healthy balance; where you are able to take care of yourself and balance that with taking care of others. Let your veganism be a reminder that self-care is important.

LOWER EXPECTATIONS THAT OTHERS WHO ARE PREPARING FOOD DURING A HEALTH CRISIS ARE GOING TO REMEMBER THAT YOU ARE A VEGAN

We suggested earlier that your veganism may make you a target for the emotions that are being released during a health crisis. On the other hand, your veganism may simply drop off the radar of those who are preparing food. Although some families do include vegan options when they are gathered together, in times of crises, this commitment may not be as easily maintained. Lowering your expectations helps in several ways. First, you aren't left without anything to eat because you thought someone else was preparing something for you.

Second, this avoids feelings of bitterness, or of being ignored. You place what is happening in clear perspective—the health-care crisis has thrown over everyone's ability to juggle multiple needs. Your need for a vegan meal may be one of those things. Recognizing this, you will always arrive prepared.

Third, you are pleasantly surprised when your veganism is remembered.

As a crisis health-care situation evolves toward a chronic one (and with parents or other older relatives and friends it just may), and you and the other caregivers evolve a process of care, your veganism may be integrated into the response of the household. A butternut squash soup is made, some of it with vegetable broth, some without. Vegetables are set aside before butter is added. A run to the grocery store includes grabbing some frozen vegan food for you.

RAISE YOUR SELF-CARE: TAKING CARE OF YOUR VEGAN NEEDS WHILE CAREGIVING

An important aspect of your self-care is ensuring that you have healthy vegan food to eat. *Be prepared to be tired, so do work in advance.* Here are some self-care food suggestions:

- If you need to stay on short notice at the residence of a friend or relative who is not vegan, on your way there, stop at a store for some essential foods or recipe ingredients, or bring them from home. The whirlwind of a household in the midst of crisis may keep you from getting to a store for a few days.
- Likewise, bring along copies of the recipes for vegan dishes you love to prepare (comfort food, fast meals, your very own perfected recipes), or your favorite cookbook. Even though you think you know a recipe by heart, stress can knock your memory for a loop!
- When you are able to, prepare more than you need and freeze it.

- Prepare mixes for baked goods (the dry ingredients) that you can use over time.

- Use grains that cook quickly—quinoa, polenta, couscous. Cook extra quinoa and throw veggies in with it; it can be tomorrow's salad.

- Opt for convenience when you need to. Keep prepared meals and veggie burgers on hand for when you need a meal in a hurry.

- Canned chickpeas are your friends. If time allows for nothing else, you can drain the can, rinse the chickpeas, dress them up with a little salad dressing from a bottle, and eat.

- Get a jar of hoisin sauce. It is a great flavor to use when cooking quickly. Toss on cooked rice. Slather on tofu and bake. Slather on sweet potatoes and bake. Its slightly sweet flavor provides a little bit of extra comfort if you find yourself craving sugar.

- Use any of your favorite condiments—salsa, mustard, seasoned rice vinegar—to quickly dress up canned beans. Serve them over any cooked grain or as a salad on a bed of lettuce.

- Frozen vegetables are just as good for you as fresh, and are often less expensive and faster to prepare. In a pinch, canned vegetables are fine to include in meals, too. They aren't quite as good for you as frozen or fresh, but eating canned veggies is better than skipping the veggies altogether.

- Vegan soup from a can or box can provide a great starter for your own "homemade" recipe. Add beans, diced cooked potatoes, and veggies and heat it up for ultimate convenience with your own special touch.

- If you are a long-term caregiver, try to get a slow cooker. It can do the cooking while you are resting. Cooking in one dish means less to clean up.

When people ask you how they can help, believe that they are earnest in their offer and give them specific suggestions. It may be that what you most need is for someone to come and give you a two-hour break. Say that. Or you may have been able to keep up with cooking for the care receiver, but you feel that you are subsisting on peanut butter and jelly sandwiches (and chickpeas!). Ask for help: could someone bring a couple of meals for the individual you are caring for? This would free up your time to fix something you need to eat. Or, if you know that the person who is offering would be happy to prepare you a vegan meal, don't be shy. Answer, "I am able to keep up with meals for Mom; what I really need is a couple of meals that could tide me over." You might make suggestions. Or ask the person to do a shopping trip for you, and explain where to find any "strange" items on your list (such as tofu, almond milk, or vegan vegetable stock). The good news is that so many grocery stores now carry these items.

FOODS THAT ARE GOOD FOR STRESS

With stress you may feel more irritable, suffer more headaches, and find your shoulders sore and your neck tight.

- Certain nutrients help your brain produce serotonin, a neurotransmitter that helps relieve stress and depression. Protein-rich foods provide tryptophan, an amino acid that is needed to make serotonin. Carbohydrates are needed to help tryptophan pass from the blood into brain cells. Beans may very well be the ultimate serotonin-boosting comfort food since they are among the only foods that are rich in both protein and carbohydrates. Use them in foods that you find soothing—baked beans or warm lentil soup can be made ahead and frozen.

- A peanut butter sandwich with fruit spread or sliced bananas is another protein-carbohydrate combo comfort food. Quinoa topped with cashew cream sauce, or barbecued tempeh over brown rice are other good choices.

- Many herbs have been used for centuries to sooth anxiety and stress. Sip teas made from catnip, valerian root, chamomile, or lemon balm.

- Although it may feel tempting to reach for sweets—and sometimes a treat may in fact be exactly what you need— try to choose more "slow carbs"—carbohydrate-rich foods that are digested and absorbed more slowly. Sweet potatoes, quinoa, barley, oats, pasta, and beans are better choices than white rice and white potatoes. They help prevent fluctuations in blood glucose that can raise risk for chronic disease.
- Make sure you're taking daily supplements of vitamin B_{12}, vitamin D, and DHA (from microalgae). A shortfall of any of these nutrients can result in feelings of depression.

IF YOU ARE THE CARE RECEIVER

IS THERE A SOCIAL STIGMA FOR VEGANS WHO GET ILL?

If you get ill, along with sympathy may come cluck-clucking. Because veganism has become associated with healthy living, vegans who become ill often find that there is a sense of shame associated with their getting sick, as though vegans shouldn't get sick.

We need to identify and understand this undeserved stigma so that it doesn't keep you from getting the help you might need.

If, as a vegan, you have health challenges, don't presume that veganism is a magic bullet that can take care of all things. This book was prompted when a discussion of dairy on Carol's Facebook page led to the admission by two women that they both had osteoporosis and had been long-time vegans.

This prompted the question, Who is talking about veganism and aging in a way that is helpful and accurate?

Because veganism is promoted as a healthful diet, vegans bear a difficult burden: Does their illness announce the failure of veganism as a healthy diet? Vegans become afraid of getting sick, because it is bad for veganism. Individual vegans are seen to be representative of the entire diet. Nonvegans may take your health issue as proof that indeed one *does* need meat or dairy or eggs. Vegans report to us, "Whenever I get a cold someone says, 'Oh you need some meat.'"

Or vegans, upon discovering that they have high blood pressure or high cholesterol, may worry, "How embarrassing if I died from a heart attack." Or they may think, "I don't want to be one of the people of whom people say, 'She did everything right, she exercised, she followed a vegan diet, and yet look at her . . .'"

We do our best not to get sick, but there are no guarantees in this world. If we are making choices out of kindness and we still get sick, it's not our fault. If we have health needs, we still need to be smart and get the help we need. No matter our diagnosis, a vegan diet gives us a foundation with which to deal with it.

VEGAN MEAL ARRANGEMENTS

Showing appreciation and being clear in expressing our needs are vitally important if we are the people receiving care.

If you are hospitalized or know you will be, appoint someone who will be your advocate to represent your needs to the medical staff. This person should be especially alert to your vegan dietary needs.

> *"I am a home health-care provider and I took care of a man who basically couldn't move or talk—he did have some movement but not much. He was a strict vegan and gluten-free. Through his form of communicating he would direct us on how he wanted us to cook, what he wanted for meals, and so on. He was the one that tasted the food while it was cooking, and then when it was done he always had us take a bite to see if we liked it. Many of his dishes were out of this world—he could have been a chef!"* —CAROL

If you are at home, there may be someone who volunteers to oversee meals for you. If not, you can ask someone to do it. As the coordinator of meals, this person should be explicit about what it is you don't eat (reminding people about chicken stock, or meat or cheese in tomato sauce, or eggs as binders in baked goods). People who want to help you recuperate will appreciate gentle but firm reminders.

If you anticipate a recuperation time, you might line up some meals in your freezer. Or make a list of local restaurants and what their vegan take-out offerings are. If you have the funds, you might be able to hire a local vegan to prepare some meals for you. You might have noticed someone whose contributions to vegan potlucks always received compliments; that person might be thrilled to be hired. It's worth a call or e-mail to find out.

A VEGAN PROTEIN/CALORIE DRINK FROM THE VEGETARIAN RESOURCE GROUP

Anyone familiar with caregiving knows the word "Ensure." Often recommended by doctors to be sure that the elderly are getting enough protein and other nutrients, it is not vegan. At one time, Westsoy offered a vegan equivalent. Two interns at the Vegetarian Resource Group, Monica Cohen and Heather Fliehman, developed a vegan version they call a "Protein/Calorie Drink."

This recipe offers as an option using a powder made from the açai berry. Açai powder packets are available from several manufacturers. They can be purchased at natural foods or grocery stores and from online vitamin stores. The açai contributes very little in terms of flavor, but it does provide some calories. Therefore, you may want to include it in the recipe.

▶ MAKES ABOUT 2 CUPS (16 OUNCES)

1 cup hemp milk (look for a brand that is fortified with vitamin B_{12})
3 ounces silken tofu, or 6 ounces mixed berry soy yogurt
1 cup fresh or frozen blueberries
One 3.5-ounce packet açai powder, optional
1 medium banana or 1 tablespoon orange juice concentrate

1. Place all the ingredients in a blender and blend until smooth.

NOTE: In comparison to Ensure, this vegan supplement does not meet all micronutrient needs. These nutrients may be obtained from other foods or, if the appetite is poor or food choices are limited, from a multivitamin/mineral supplement. Also, nut butters are frequently good sources of vitamin E and zinc. Please consult with your health-care provider, concerning what is appropriate for you. Source: vrg.org/journal/vj2009issue2/2009_issue2_supplement.php.

VEGANS OVER 50 TELL THEIR STORIES

A Mom Moves to Assisted Living | Roni Omohundro

Roni's story: Roni Omohundro became a vegan when she was fifty-three. Her daughter, Jasmin, had become a vegan and was doing activist work around animal issues. (Jasmin is the co-founder of OurHenHouse.org, an online nonprofit multimedia hub of opportunities to change the world for animals.)

Roni had been suffering from migraine headaches and also felt she had some eating disorder issues. She decided she wanted to try Jasmin's lifestyle for three weeks. That was nine years ago, and she's been a vegan ever since.

Roni now keeps a vegan home. For almost a year, her own eighty-eight-year-old mom, Sherrey Reim Glickman, lived with Roni and her husband. (Sherrey's story can be found on page 34.) "She ate really well when she ate with me," said Roni. Sherrey liked the substitutes, "such as making a chickpea salad taste like a tuna salad." Sometimes she would watch Roni prepare the food, or help prep the vegetables. Sherrey also accompanied Roni when she went food shopping.

Roni reported, "When my mom was at home with me, she lived in an environment of veganism—not just eating, but discussing it. My mom had been an activist, and these vegan ideas appealed to her as an activist."

Sherrey developed a brain tumor that contributed to a lack of mobility. When it got to the point where she couldn't stand up on her own, she needed more professional help than Roni could provide.

In 2013, Sherrey moved to assisted living. And then the challenges began. As Roni explains, "We have been having a hard time getting her appropriate food. I talked to the head of the food service who said they could do veggie burgers. They could also do wraps with beans and rice, pizza, salad, soups. That's pretty much it. They don't get into the greens. Their greens are broccoli and some greens in soups. The salads are pretty simple—lettuce and tomato, pretty much standard fare.

"I am disappointed. We were not able to find an assisted living facility near us that offers vegan/vegetarian food as an option."

WORKING WITH RETIREMENT COMMUNITIES, ASSISTED LIVING CENTERS, AND NURSING HOMES

Let's face it: vegans can end up in assisted living centers and nursing homes. Our diet may reduce the risk that we'll develop chronic diseases and perhaps can even give some protection against Alzheimer's disease. But even vegans can become ill or develop conditions that no longer allow us to care for ourselves. We aren't alone in thinking, "If I ever get dementia, I still want to be a vegan."

How do we work with institutions for the aging population to increase vegan options?

Debra Wasserman and Charles Stahler, Coordinators of the Vegetarian Resource Group, recount the experience of Ed Murphy:

The [assisted living] facility where he lives was already serving some items that he was able to eat, including baked potatoes, prunes, bananas, an assortment of cereal, juice, tossed salad, beets, and cabbage slaw with pepper (instead of mayonnaise). Ed bought soy milk from a local supermarket, which is much easier today than even a few years ago.

For breakfast, Ed just wanted simple items. For other meals, food service did offer some vegetarian entrées, like spaghetti with tomato sauce. They also tried to accommodate his special needs by serving items such as veggie burgers purchased from the local supermarket. Ed put some lettuce and onion on the burger, which is usually served with a side of carrots, vegetarian baked beans, lima beans, and green beans. However, he admits he was getting a little tired of eating them. "Everyone thinks you want veggie burgers every night," Ed said. "It's kind of like eating a hamburger every night."

We talked with Dr. Neal Barnard, president of Physicians Committee for Responsible Medicine (PCRM). PCRM has developed menu resources for large institutions and has helped businesses and schools adopt vegan meal plans. But Dr. Barnard observed that working with retirement communities requires an additional step. "If you just offered a vegan meal in a nursing home it would fall flat."

Dr. Barnard has recommended a two-pronged approach: advocating with the administration to include more vegan foods and making sure the population is educated and asking for these foods. "Talk to a group of residents. Ask, 'How many of you are on medications?' Describe how nutrition could help their diabetes and reduce their medication needs." Dr. Barnard continued, "This is a highly motivated group. I hear that people who are old don't want to change. People rattle that off all the time. But it's not true. If people feel that their health is involved, they do change. This is the group with more risk of Alzheimer's, diabetes, heart disease. They often are on a boatload of medications that cause a lot of complications as well as being expensive. They might not know there is an alternative."

Dr. Barnard observed that when you are sixteen or twenty-six, these health concerns are hypothetical issues. But when you are sixty, or seventy, or eighty, these health issues are very real. When he talks to older people, he says, "How many of you would want to reduce your reliance on your medications? What if one of the choices you had every day here was a completely vegan meal, like veggie chili or spaghetti marinara?" Barnard pointed out that providing taste tests is really important; people form their opinions about what they like to eat very early in life and they need an opportunity to learn about new foods, rather than having them simply appear on the menu.

Education builds demand, and demand creates opportunity. Perhaps local vegan groups could adopt retirement homes in their community and provide education. Or perhaps vegan high school students could get credit for their required community service by devising an education program for assisted living, drawing on such resources as DVDs.

SELECTING A RETIREMENT COMMUNITY

We know that more than anything, geography may determine your decision as to where to move. Where you want to live, or who you want to live near, are often the most important factors.

Learn whether the place you're considering serves any kinds of vegan food. One director of dining in a retirement community with whom we spoke observed, "For the most part, our group, up to the last five years, was primarily the meat and potatoes group. Fresh produce and fresh fish were always available. We are seeing, as in the general population, people seeking out more local and fresh foods." Is this true for the facility you are considering?

Find out whether there is a residents' committee that works with the director of dining. If so, what has it tackled in the past? If not, would such a committee be considered?

Is the independent living residence dining plan a strict one or is it a flex dining plan?

In the ideal situation, veganism would be considered like other special requests (such as diabetic or gluten-free), and the needed products would be available. One Quaker retirement home makes casseroles using quinoa, couscous, and bulgur wheat. It also prepares vegetable stir-fries. If they are making eggplant Parmesan, they might do ratatouille for the vegan, keeping the element of the eggplant in the dish, but not the cheese. In addition to the scheduled menu of the day and the vegetarian and vegan items of the day, they have a selection of "always available food items," including hummus. Because of different food allergies, they list every ingredient on the menu. This ideal situation is not found in all places, at least, not yet.

Expanding Meal Options

If you are in assisted living or a nursing home, make sure that you or your family members advocate for you, working with the administration or a staff dietitian to create more options for you as a vegan. Many who are responsible for the menus at these facilities may not even realize that vegan products are readily available. For example, Sysco, one of the largest food vendors supplying schools, skilled nursing facilities, and group homes, offers vegan cookies, veggie meat mixes, and even vegan cheeses.

If you are the only vegan in residence, kitchen staff may welcome ideas for very simple vegan meals, or meals that can easily be veganized. Pasta with spaghetti sauce is one meal that can go either way. It can be topped with meatballs for meat eaters, and sautéed white beans with onions for your vegan meal. Lentil soup seasoned with liquid smoke is likely to appeal to both vegans and meat eaters.

Don't hesitate to suggest some more interesting vegan meals, though. You might share a copy of the cookbook *Vegan in Volume* by Chef Nancy Berkoff with the dietitian or food service director. It provides instructions for preparing vegan meals for large groups with tips on menus for retirement homes.

If all else fails, family members could bring in food items. Perhaps someone can help you create and cook foods in your actual unit.

• • •

Whenever and however you are called upon to be a caregiver, we hope that the suggestions in this chapter will help you meet the challenges and take comfort in the blessings that come with aiding another in need. If you take away nothing else, try to remember our guidelines for vegan caregiving: Lower your expectations, raise your self-care, protect the boundaries you can, and enjoy healthy vegan meals.

We wish you ease and well-being as you share your heart, time, and energy with those you care for.

PART FOUR

LET'S EAT!

D ID YOU SKIP to this part first? Many people want to know what's cooking and can't wait to see the recipes and a discussion of food.

Or maybe you postponed coming to this part. Vegans are diverse and have different priorities and needs. For many, food preparation, vegan or not, is a chore and there are all kinds of things they would rather be doing—and that's perfectly okay. We want to provide options for those who love to cook (or who might rediscover a love of cooking when they go vegan), but we don't imagine that just because you go vegan, you will become an avid cook if you weren't before.

We have recipes, meal ideas, and suggestions for all kinds of cooks.

If you are still working your way through the maze of how to live without basic dairy products or eggs, head to chapter 10, "How to Veganize."

If you're just learning to cook, we have many easy recipes to help you find your footing. We also offer variations for these recipes; for instance, Roasted Vegetables (page 280): one day you may want to roast Brussels sprouts; another day, carrots or green beans. Once you learn the technique, the difference is in the seasonings and the time it takes for a vegetable to roast. We also provide several options for cooking grains and beans. We'll teach you how to scramble tofu and fry foods with a vegan batter.

If recipes aren't your thing at all, or you're an experimental cook, take a look at pages 267–270, where we give suggestions for vegan meals that don't require recipes or any particular cooking skill. We've also created a chart on page 213 to provide some guidance on "mixing and matching" foods and leftovers to build fast healthy meals.

No matter what your relationship to preparing food has been in the past, you will find resources here to help you with your next step.

> **SOME COMMERCIAL BREADS AND** crackers contain animal ingredients. A quick scan of the nutrition label—particularly the list of potential allergens at the end of the ingredient list—will alert you to products that are not vegan. Watch for added whey, milk powder, cheese, and eggs.

We have collected recipes and tips from a variety of sources, including some of the vegans whose stories you have read earlier in the book. Donald Moy (page 180) described how he loved his mom's vegan macaroni and cheese; we asked whether we could reprint it so others, too, could enjoy it (page 302). Colleen Welsh (page 15) discovered that she loved to veganize her grandmother's recipes. We asked her for a few of her favorites and she sent us "Chicken" Piccata (page 301) and Beans and Greens (page 299). After trying commercial seitan, Sandy Weiland (page 158) experimented with making her own seitan and came up with her own meat substitute (page 231) so that she could continue to use her favorite meat recipes. In the next chapter, you will learn how Christina Nakhoda (page 226) began veganizing baked goods for her vegan and vegetarian children. How could we not collect a couple of her favorite recipes to share (pages 297, 318 and 321)?

Patti, Carol, and Ginny each developed vegan cooking styles based on factors having to do with individual habits and interests. As longtime vegans, we have each developed a list of go-to recipes that work for us. We have also been fortunate to have vegan recipe innovators as friends.

In the mid-1980s, vegan cookbooks were few and hard to find. During the first few years that they were vegan, both Carol and Patti independently purchased a copy of every vegan cookbook in print. Yet they each gravitated to Jennifer Raymond's *Peaceful Palate* as the basis for many of their favorite meals. (Raymond has graciously given permission for many of these favorites to be featured in the recipe section). The late Shirley Wilkes-Johnson, a close friend of Carol's and an excellent vegan chef and teacher, was the original source of some of the recipes we're delighted to be able to share with you. Shirley taught vegan cooking classes in the Houston area for many years. She also loved veganizing favorite Texas recipes (as an example of such a recipe, see her Corny Dogs, page 309).

OUR VEGAN LIVES

Our Favorite Cooking Resources

Patti:

> *Eat Vegan on $4 a Day* by Ellen Jaffe Jones
> *Main Street Vegan* by Victoria Moran
> Vegkitchen.com, author Nava Atlas's website
> the recipes at ForksOverKnives.com

Carol: At this point in time, new vegan cookbooks are being published every month, and it seems impossible to keep up with all of them. But I try; I probably own over five hundred vegan and vegetarian cookbooks. I love reading them. I find myself intellectually stimulated by the plant-based combinations vegan chefs come up with. I like learning new approaches to menus. I find both a freedom and a fantasy in reading vegan cookbooks. Even though I know there are some recipes I will never actually fix, I feel a sense of happiness that vegan chefs are helping create such luscious meals.

I also check out new posts on various websites, including:

> theppk.com/recipes
> Veganyumyum.com
> Compassionatecooks.com
> Fatfreevegan.com
> Ohsheglows.com
> Vegandad.blogspot.com

Ginny: Although I still use tried-and-true recipes from my early days as a vegan, there is a new generation of books by cooks who have taken vegan cooking to a whole new level. These are some of my favorites:

Big Vegan by Robin Asbell

Blissful Bites by Christy Morgan

The Blooming Platter by Betsy DiJulio

Let Them Eat Vegan by Dreena Burton

Tofu Cookery, 25th Anniversary Edition by Louise Hagler

The Urban Vegan by Dynise Balcavage

Quick and Easy Vegan Comfort Food by Alicia Simpson

Vegan Diner by Julie Hasson

Vegan Eats World by Terry Hope Romero

Vegan on the Cheap by Robin Robertson

Vegan Brunch by Isa Chandra Moskowitz

World Vegan Feast by Bryanna Clark Grogan

Some of my favorite blogs for finding great vegan recipes include:

JLGoesVegan.com

thevword.net

theppk.com

francostigan.com/recipes.html (for decadent vegan desserts)

I also follow all of these inspired cooks—the bloggers and the cookbook writers—on Pinterest, which keeps me happily up to my ears in great vegan recipes.

APPLIANCES FOR A VEGAN KITCHEN

These appliances, if you already have them in your kitchen, are great for vegan cooking and baking:

- a food processor equipped with an "S" steel blade
- a blender, for smoothies and soups
- an immersion blender, for soups
- a handheld mixer, for batter and frosting
- a cast-iron skillet

- a George Foreman grill, for tofu, tempeh, or veggie hot dogs
- a bread baker (Substitute soy milk or almond milk if your bread recipe calls for milk.)
- a slow cooker, (for beans, chilis, and stews)
- a rice cooker (Quinoa cooks beautifully in a rice cooker.)
- a pressure cooker (Beans in 10 minutes!)

FOOD PREPARATION UTENSILS AND EQUIPMENT

- a tofu press (TofuXpress is the manufacturer of this helpful kitchen implement, which does all the work of expressing water out of tofu.)
- a fine-mesh strainer, for rinsing quinoa and rice
- a jelly-roll pan (15 × 10 inches with 1-inch sides) for Mom's Vegan Cinnamon Rolls (page 318) and the Texas Sheet Cake (page 323)
- a 9 × 5-inch loaf pan, for the Mushroom Pâté (page 274) and Neatloaf (page 310)
- a steamer, for making the Vegan Meat (seitan) (page 231) and for steaming veggies
- cheesecloth
- butcher string, for vegan sausage and vegan meat recipes
- parchment paper

HOW TO BUILD A HEALTHY VEGAN MEAL

When you have a well-stocked pantry, refrigerator and freezer, dinner comes together with little effort or planning. You can use recipes or not, depending on how much time and effort you want to put into meal preparation.

Start with a foundation of vegetables and add whole grains or potatoes, plus some type of legume. Top it with a savory sauce (you can even use your favorite soup!) or a sprinkle of crunchy nuts or a drizzle of some type of flavorful condiment.

Mix and match from the following chart to put together a variety of healthy and interesting meals. (You don't need to use choices from all four columns for every meal; it's all about what works for you.)

EASY VEGAN MEAL IDEAS

- brown basmati rice; shredded cabbage and tofu sautéed in olive oil; a sprinkle of toasted sesame seeds
- pasta tossed with sautéed carrots, zucchini, peas, and slices of Tofurky Italian sausage and topped with vegan Parmesan cheese
- pasta and steamed broccoli topped with textured vegetable protein cooked in vegan tomato sauce
- baked sweet potatoes on a bed of steamed collards served with Indonesian Peanut Sauce (page 304)
- baked white potatoes stuffed with steamed broccoli and cauliflower and homemade Vegan Feta Cheese (page 222)
- brown rice; cabbage, peppers, bok choy, and tofu stir-fried in toasted sesame oil and seasoned with seasoned rice vinegar and fresh ginger
- brown rice; black beans, salsa, and guacamole with a big topping of shredded lettuce and chopped tomatoes
- baked potato topped with Red Lentil Soup with Curry (page 272); Confetti Slaw (page 258)
- quinoa, corn, and canned pinto beans tossed with chopped raw onions, celery, and Yogurt-Tahini Dressing (page 255); steamed Brussels sprouts
- braised collards, corn bread, canned black-eyed peas with smoky Soy Curls (see page 232)
- raw vegetables topped with hummus; baked sweet potato with a sprinkle of balsamic vinegar
- Scrambled Tofu (page 245) with vegan cheese rolled into a whole wheat tortilla or stuffed in a pita pocket; salad with dressing.

HOW TO BUILD A HEALTHY VEGAN MEAL

	START WITH A MOUNTAIN OF VEGETABLES—AS MANY DIFFERENT ONES AS YOU LIKE	ADD WHOLE GRAINS OR POTATOES	INCLUDE SOME PROTEIN-PACKED LEGUMES	EMBELLISH WITH A SAVORY SAUCE OR SOMETHING TO ADD A LITTLE CRUNCH OR UMAMI
When you need to keep it simple	Plain steamed or sautéed vegetables, such as broccoli, cauliflower, bok choy, Brussels sprouts, cabbage (red, green, Napa), carrots, peas, kale, collards, beet greens, chard, spinach, beets, zucchini, corn, green beans Raw chopped tomatoes, peppers, or shredded carrots, cabbage, lettuce	Pasta Baked or steamed yams, sweet potatoes, or white potatoes Brown rice, barley, quinoa, or kasha (buckwheat groats) Whole-grain vegan bread or tortillas	Canned or home-cooked beans (black, navy, pinto, black-eyed peas, adzuki, kidney) Steamed tempeh Prepared seitan or baked tofu Veggie meats	Toasted seeds (pumpkin, sesame, sunflower) Chopped nuts (walnuts, almonds, hazelnuts, cashews, pecans, pistachios) Guacamole or avocado slices Seasoned rice vinegar Balsamic vinegar Vegan tomato or Sloppy Joe sauce from a jar Vegan shredded cheese Mirin (sweet Japanese cooking wine) Any favorite salad dressing
When you feel like cooking	Roasted Vegetables (page 280) Spicy Collards with Ginger (page 282) Kale with Cinnamon (page 283) Greens and Mushrooms (page 284) Massaged Kale Salad (page 260) Confetti Slaw (page 258)	Festive Quinoa (page 297) Minted Barley Salad (page 262)	Soy Curls (page 232) Fast, Filling Chili (page 273) Basic Hummus (page 249) Scrambled Tofu (page 245) Sweet and Spicy Baked Tofu (page 307)	Indonesian Peanut Sauce (page 304) Vegan Feta Cheese (page 222) Vegan Parmesan (page 224) Yogurt-Tahini Dressing (page 255) White Bean Gravy with Ginger and Cinnamon (page 286) Red Lentil Soup with Curry (page 272)

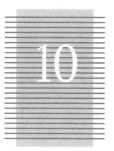

10

HOW TO VEGANIZE:
BASIC SUBSTITUTIONS

RECIPES IN THIS CHAPTER

Holiday Nog
Tofu Sour Cream
Vegan Feta/Cottage Cheese
Tofu Ricotta Cheese
Vegan Parmesan
Dragonfly's Bulk Dry Uncheese Mix
Vegan Mayo
Vegan Sausage and Vegan Meat (Seitan)
Vegan "Pulled Pork"
Dolphin- and Tuna-Friendly Mork-Tuna Salad

FOR SOME OF US, there isn't a traditional dish that we can't make vegan. You may remember the artichoke appetizer that was ubiquitous in the 1970s, which was heavy on mayonnaise and Parmesan cheese. Even that can be veganized (see page 224).

At this point, people have been veganizing for decades, and none of us has to invent new ways of doing this. That doesn't mean that some of us don't want to tackle the challenge. A few years ago, Carol tried but failed to veganize brioche, which in its traditional version is rich in both eggs and butter. (She no longer remembers just why it was that she wanted to try to do this—probably just for the challenge.) Now, several vegan brioche recipes can be found (and there is an entire cookbook on how to prepare vegan French baked goods, The Vegan Boulangerie, which, yes, includes a brioche recipe).

Does veganizing mean you have to throw out everything in your pantry and start all over? No. Peek into a vegan pantry and you may find that it looks just like yours or your mom's. Rice, pasta, spaghetti sauce, canned tomatoes, ketchup, and mustard are all staples in many vegan kitchens, and some vegans never venture too far from the ingredients they grew up with. But part of the fun of a vegan diet is in exploring new foods and veganizing old favorites. There are so many wonderful products and ingredients that make vegan cooking and eating easier and more interesting than ever. You'll find that your pantry may soon contain vegan Worcestershire sauce (traditionally made with anchovies) or vegetable broth powder or soup stock.

Does veganizing mean you have to use tofu? No. Many people, especially many over age fifty, associate tofu with its emergence as a food of choice for vegetarians in the 1970s. Granted, at that time there were some uninspired ways of preparing tofu. But not anymore. Vegan cooking—with or without tofu—has emerged as a creative and varied cuisine. Use tofu when you want and don't use it when you don't want. Tofu is to the cook what an empty canvas is to an artist.

Tofu is often used to create vegan versions of dairy foods, such as sour cream, ranch dressing, Caesar dressing, feta cheese, and ricotta cheese. It is made in the same way that cheese is made from cow's milk: a curdling agent is added to soy milk. Throughout Asia, tofu is made fresh daily from soybeans in small shops and sold on the street by vendors. If you are stir-frying chunks of tofu with veggies to serve over rice, choose firm tofu. For dishes that call for pureed tofu—say, a pâté or dip, soft tofu is the best choice. And the tofu that is traditional to Japanese cooking, silken tofu, is a soft custard-like food that can be blended or pureed for sauces, smoothies, and desserts. It makes a great replacement for the cream in creamed soup recipes. At many supermarkets, you'll also find seasoned baked or smoked tofu that is ready to heat and eat.

Pressing tofu to remove excess water improves its texture and also its ability to absorb other flavors in a dish. In the past, the only way to do this was to wrap the tofu in paper towels and then place it under a plate weighted by something heavy, such as a large can of beans. Now you can purchase a tofu press that does the work for you. You'll also discover that freezing tofu, defrosting it, and wringing out excess liquid changes the texture, making it especially porous and spongy.

We'll give you lots of options in this chapter, because as we said at the beginning of this book, people become vegans and live as vegans in their own way.

> "I wish I had known how good I would feel, physically and mentally. I also wish I had known how much fun it would be to cook vegan. I've always enjoyed cooking, but my interest in it and enthusiasm for it has increased tenfold since I became vegan." —LINDA

MILK FROM PLANTS

You'll find fortified plant-based milks made from rice, almonds, soybeans, hemp seeds, and coconut in the refrigerated section of stores and also packaged aseptically. These are usually interchangeable in recipes. Look for brands that are fortified with calcium and vitamin D. (Canned coconut milk is not the coconut milk being sold in the refrigerator section. Canned coconut milk is the liquid produced from grated, fresh coconut. It is high in saturated fat, so look for reduced-fat coconut milk in the international foods section of the grocery store. You'll see that it is popular in Thai and Indian recipes.)

How do you decide which plant-based milk to use? Have a milk tasting (see page 33).

When using a plant-based milk for cooking, use unsweetened milk for savory foods, but vanilla-flavored milk is fine for most baking.

OTHER DAIRY SUBSTITUTES

VEGAN YOGURT

Found in most natural foods stores, vegan yogurt is made from soy, almond, or coconut milk and is a good source of probiotics. Read the ingredients label carefully to ensure the product is totally vegan.

VEGAN BUTTERMILK

It's easy to make your own vegan buttermilk. Just put 1 tablespoon of cider vinegar or fresh lemon juice in a glass measuring cup (do not use a metal container) and fill with unsweetened soy milk to the one-cup level. Let stand for 10 minutes so that it separates. (We use soy milk because it clabbers better than other plant-based milks.)

VEGAN "EGG" NOG

You can purchase vegan "nogs" around the holidays. Look for So Delicious brand coconut milk nog or Silk brand Soy Nog. Or you can make your own.

HOLIDAY NOG

This traditional favorite is great with or without the alcohol. Serve it in wine glasses for a clinking toast to good health.

▶ **SERVES 4**

1 quart soy milk
6 ounces silken tofu
6 tablespoons pure maple syrup
2 teaspoons pure vanilla extract
1½ teaspoons ground cardamom
½ teaspoon freshly grated nutmeg
¼ teaspoon ground cloves
¼ cup brandy or amaretto, optional

1. Blend all the ingredients in a blender and chill.

"My family has always enjoyed a large punchbowl full of egg nog on Christmas Eve. I stopped drinking it, of course, when I became vegan. Then I discovered store-bought vegan nog. Love it! Now I don't have to buy commercial vegan nog because I can make my own from scratch."
—SUSAN

VEGAN SOUR CREAM

Commercial brands of vegan sour cream are usually made with a tofu base. Tofutti and Follow Your Heart are two widely available brands. You can also make your own.

TOFU SOUR CREAM

▶ **MAKES 1½ CUPS**

One 12-ounce package silken (soft) tofu
2½ tablespoons fresh lemon juice
2½ teaspoons sugar
¼ teaspoon salt

1. Combine all the ingredients in a food processor and process until smooth. Chill for at least 2 hours to allow the flavors to blend. Stored in the refrigerator, this will keep for about 2 weeks.

VEGAN CREAM OR WHIPPED CREAM

Several brands of nondairy cream are available commercially, such as MimiCreme, a sweetened whippable cream made from nuts. You can also make a cashew cream by soaking raw cashews in water for several hours or overnight. Drain the cashews and puree in a food processor, adding water to achieve the desired consistency. Some people add a couple of teaspoons of any liquid sweetener.

WHIPPED COCONUT CREAM

TO GET A WHIPPABLE cream, refrigerate one can of coconut milk. The next day, without tipping the can, scoop out the solidified top and beat it with a mixer for 30 seconds. Beat in ¼ cup of confectioners' sugar and 1 teaspoon of vanilla. Vegan cooks then have a choice: whip until frothy and serve, or whip the coconut mixture for just 10 seconds. Refrigerate it for about an hour, then using a whisk, beat it until all the lumps disappear, and serve. Makes about 1 cup.

If you love whipped sweet potatoes, whip them with coconut milk instead of heavy cream.

VEGAN BUTTER

Instead of dairy butter, use vegan margarine, often carried in the refrigerator case right alongside the dairy butters in grocery and natural foods stores. You can also make your own (several good recipes are on the Internet). On toast, you can skip the margarine and use hummus, apple butter, pear butter, mashed avocado, nut butters or seed butters. On sweet potatoes, try a little hoisin sauce, Cranberry Fig Relish (page 254), or leftover soup.

VEGAN ICE CREAM

You'll find lots of vegan ice creams, made from soy, coconut, cashew, rice, hemp seed, and almond milks, in the freezer section of natural foods and grocery stores. Read the ingredients label of ices and sorbets to ensure that they are totally vegan.

THE WORLD OF VEGAN CHEESES

So what to do about cheese? A variety of nondairy cheeses are made from soy, almonds, or rice (read the label carefully to ensure that they do not contain casein, a milk protein). Look for vegan Jack-, Cheddar-, or mozzarella-style cheese, including prepared vegan cheese slices or "meltable" shreds (we recommend Daiya brand), and grated Parmesan-style cheese. Vegan cream cheese is also available in small tubs.

You can also make your own cheese. You'll find everything from Velveeta-like cheese spread to Brie in the *The Ultimate UnCheese Cookbook* by Jo Stepaniak, *The Cheesy Vegan* by John Schlimm, and *Artisan Vegan Cheese* by Miyoko Schinner.

For many cheeses, you will most likely need to get to know nutritional yeast, a flaked or powdered condiment that gives foods a cheesy flavor and is a popular item in many veganized foods. Look for Red Star brand Vegetarian Support Formula because it provides vitamin B_{12}. It also keeps for a long time, so don't hesitate to buy more than your recipe calls for.

VEGAN FETA/COTTAGE CHEESE

The late Shirley Wilkes-Johnson, who was Carol's friend and an extraordinary vegan chef, created this recipe for the "Celebrate Greece" class that she taught in Houston, and her students went wild over it. Use this creamy vegan version of feta cheese in a Greek salad or any salad, or in a Greek pizza or any pizza. Spread it on crackers or mix some of it with guacamole. This can also be used in place of ricotta or cottage cheese.

▶ MAKES 1½ POUNDS (3 CUPS)

1 pound extra-firm tofu
One 8-ounce package nondairy cream cheese, preferably Tofutti
    Better Than Cream Cheese (see note)
¼ cup extra virgin olive oil (preferably Greek)
¼ cup fresh lemon juice
2 teaspoons salt
½ teaspoon garlic powder

1. Rinse the tofu and pat it dry. Then crumble it slightly into a bowl. Use a tablespoon to add the Tofutti cream cheese, and mix in the remaining ingredients with a fork. Do not overmix. It should appear chunky and crumbly. Store covered, in the refrigerator. Use within a week's time.

NOTE: If you don't have the Tofutti cream cheese, you can leave it out and still achieve the result of a great feta-style cheese. It won't be as creamy. What people love about feta cheese is the salt and the fat. With the ingredients we substitute here, this recipe provides both.

VARIATIONS: Add some or all of these fresh herbs: garlic, crushed; parsley; dill; chives or scallions. You can also add freshly ground black or white pepper, or red pepper flakes.

TOFU RICOTTA CHEESE

This luscious "ricotta" is ideal with lasagna, ravioli, or stuffed shells, and it can even be used as a dip. Patti likes to serve this cheese when entertaining nonvegan friends and has seen how much they enjoy it.

▶ MAKES ABOUT 2 CUPS (ENOUGH TO FILL ONE SMALL CASSEROLE FOR LASAGNA)

1 pound firm or extra-firm tofu, pressed
2 tablespoons fresh lemon juice
3 tablespoons extra virgin olive oil
½ teaspoon salt
2 garlic cloves, peeled
1 teaspoon mellow barley miso
1 tablespoon finely chopped fresh rosemary

1. Process the tofu, lemon juice, oil, salt, garlic, and miso in a food processor fitted with a metal "S" blade. Stop a few times during the processing to scrape the ingredients from the sides of the processor bowl. Continue processing until the tofu has a smooth but slightly granular texture.
2. Add the rosemary and pulse to combine. Refrigerate until ready to use.

VEGAN PARMESAN

It is easy to make your own Parmesan cheese substitute.

Almond meal (see note)
Nutritional yeast
Onion powder, optional
Salt, optional

1. Mix equal amounts of almond meal and nutritional yeast together in a jar. Shake well, add a small amount of onion powder and salt, if desired, shake again, and it's ready. Store in the refrigerator until ready to use.

NOTE: Prepared almond meal is available commercially, in natural foods stores or the gluten-free baking section of grocery stores. Or make your own by pulsing raw almonds in a food processor until very finely ground. (Be sure not to overprocess or you will end up with almond butter instead of almond meal.) Store almond meal in the freezer until needed.

DRAGONFLY'S BULK DRY UNCHEESE MIX

Everyone we know swears by this. You can pour it over veggies, use it on pasta, and even make a vegan grilled cheese sandwich with it.

▶ MAKES ABOUT 6 CUPS (ENOUGH FOR 24 INDIVIDUAL SERVINGS)

3 cups raw, organic cashew pieces
2 cups nutritional yeast
3 tablespoons seasoning salt
3 tablespoons garlic powder (not garlic salt)
3 tablespoons onion powder (not onion salt)
½ cup arrowroot powder (see note)

1. Using a very dry blender or food processor, pulse the nuts until they are very fine. (Be careful not to overprocess, or you'll end up with cashew butter.)

2. Transfer to a dry bowl, add the remaining ingredients, and pulse in batches of about 1 cup.

3. Store in a dry container. This keeps in the refrigerator for 6 weeks, or in the freezer for 3 months.

4. To make sauce, combine ½ cup of the dry mix and 1 cup of water in a small saucepan. Stir over medium heat until thickened.

NOTE: You can use cornstarch, but arrowroot gives a more "stringy" cheeselike texture; chickpea flour can also be used.

GOING EGG-FREE

BAKING WITHOUT EGGS

So many ways to replace eggs exist today you don't have to abandon your favorite baked goods (including brioche!). Ener-G Egg Replacer is a widely available commercial product that you mix with water to create an egg substitute for baking. Hampton Creek Foods' Beyond Eggs for Cookies is marketed especially for baking. But you can also make your own egg replacers. You may notice many vegan recipes use vegan buttermilk (see page 218, or "Vegan Baking" below) in baked goods. The acidity in the buttermilk acts with baking soda to help baked goods expand and rise, which are functions of eggs and egg replacers in recipes. Alternatively, these each replace one egg:

1 tablespoon ground flaxseeds whisked into 3 tablespoons water; let sit until thick

1 tablespoon full-fat soy flour plus 3 tablespoons water

¼ cup soft tofu pureed with 2 teaspoons cornstarch

¼ cup applesauce plus 1 teaspoon baking powder
¼ cup vegan yogurt

Vegan Baking

When Carol's friend Christina Nakhoda stopped by to drop off some orange scones that she and her daughter, Marria, had just made, Carol prevailed upon her to share her vegan baking tips. Christina loves to cook for her family. As her two college-age children and her high school-age son became more and more interested in veganism, she was worried about what to do if she stopped using eggs in her treasured recipes. An experienced home baker, she didn't want to stop preparing her family's favorite baked goods, but wondered whether vegan treats could actually pass the taste test. Carol gave her the Banana Cake recipe (page 325) and also some Ener-G Egg Replacer. The Banana Cake has remained a favorite. Then Christina decided to veganize her own recipes.

"I made the transition from butter to vegan margarine immediately and then from milk to soy milk. My biggest breakthrough was when I went online and noticed that my favorite baking recipes had already been veganized. That was my greatest discovery, that I could bake still. I thought that baking would never be the same, but clearly it is."

She has always liked recipes that use buttermilk and sour cream because she liked the texture and taste they produced. She tried curdling soy milk with vinegar to make buttermilk, but she didn't quite get the thickness she wanted.

"Instead of using buttermilk, I have taken Tofutti sour cream and thinned it out with soy milk and that works well because that gives it a consistency like buttermilk."

Christina has found that vegan cakes in general may feel

slightly denser. She says, "It won't be the same, but it will be equally good."

That's why she believes that for a baker, simply replacing the eggs with a commercial egg replacer is not going to feel adequate. She finds that the texture of the cake isn't quite the same.

Now she prefers to let a variety of ingredients replace the egg, rather than a direct one-to-one substitution with Ener-G Egg Replacer. For instance, she will dissolve the Ener-G Egg Replacer in applesauce or mashed bananas to create a better texture.

One recipe Christina thought she'd be unable to make was cinnamon rolls. But she experimented with her mom's old recipe and it worked so well we included it in this book (page 318). She also veganized a Southern favorite, Hummingbird Cake (page 321). She'll work and rework a recipe until she feels the results are just as she remembers it.

"I thought those were recipes that were going to be only in my past, but I discovered I could re-create them." As someone who bakes for large events that include her siblings and their families, she loves when she can re-create something they have eaten for years. "I take a lot of joy in slipping [a veganized version] in and, when no one recognizes that it has changed, then I know that I have succeeded."

REPLACING EGGS IN SAVORY GOODS

When preparing vegan meat loaf or burgers, replace one egg in any recipe with ¼ cup of pumpkin puree, silken tofu, mashed beans, or mashed potatoes; 3 tablespoons of tomato paste; or 2 tablespoons of arrowroot plus 1 tablespoon water.

SWEETENERS

MANY VEGANS AVOID COMMERCIAL white sugar because it is filtered through bone char. Plenty of great vegan sweeteners are on the market including beet sugar, date sugar, rice syrup, barley malt syrup, agave syrup, and maple syrup. Organic sugar is also produced in a way that does not depend on bone char. You'll probably want to keep vegan white sugar, brown sugar, and one liquid sweetener on hand.

VEGAN MAYONNAISE

Eggless mayonnaise products include Vegenaise (Follow Your Heart), Nayonaise (Nasoya) and Mindful Mayo (Earth Balance). All are great vegan alternatives to egg-based mayonnaise. Hampton Creek Foods has also created a vegan mayonnaise, called Just Mayo, using their Beyond Egg product. You can also make your own.

VEGAN MAYO

This recipe comes from Bryanna Clark Grogan, the author of *World Vegan Feast*. Bryanna's blog, *Notes from the Vegan Feast Kitchen* (veganfeast-kitchen.blogspot.com), offers a wealth of information on the science of vegan cooking along with superb vegan recipes.

In this recipe she uses agar, which is a sea vegetable that can be used to thicken dishes. When agar powder is boiled in water, it gains a gelatin-like consistency. In fact, you can boil it in juice to create your own vegan Jell-O. You can find agar powder in natural foods stores or Asian markets. (Note: This recipe uses agar powder, not agar flakes.)

▶ MAKES 2 CUPS

1 cup any plant-based milk, such as soy or almond
2 tablespoons cider vinegar

1½ teaspoons salt

¾ teaspoon dry mustard

¼ cup extra virgin olive oil

½ teaspoon agar powder

3½ tablespoons cornstarch

1. Combine the plant-based milk, vinegar, salt, dry mustard, and olive oil in a blender and set aside.

2. In a small saucepan, combine ½ cup plus 2 tablespoons cold water and the agar powder and let stand for a few minutes. Whisk in the cornstarch until it is well combined. Cook over high heat, stirring constantly, until thick and translucent. Scrape off any cornstarch that may have stuck to the bottom, so it doesn't get left behind.

3. Add the cornstarch mixture to the other ingredients in the blender and blend until white and frothy and emulsified (which means you shouldn't see any fat globules).

4. At this point, it will look considerably thinner than regular mayonnaise, but it will thicken up as it cools. Pour into a clean jar, cover tightly, and refrigerate for several hours until set.

5. Whisk the mayo with a wire whisk (don't use a blender at this point) until it is creamy. Return to the refrigerator and let it set again.

NOTE: If you'd like a dressing that tastes more like Miracle Whip, increase the dry mustard to 1 teaspoon and add an additional tablespoon of vinegar or lemon juice plus 1 tablespoon of sugar.

REPLACING "EGGS" AS EGGS

Tofu makes a great scramble. Vegan cooks often add a pinch of ground turmeric because it gives tofu that beautiful golden color to mimic the yellow of eggs (see page 245 for our version of Scrambled Tofu). Also look online or in Indian markets for Kala Namak, or black salt. Its mineral content gives it the odor and flavor of eggs. (And it's actually pink in color.) If you want to experiment with omelets and quiches, we recommend the cookbook *Vegan Brunch* by Isa Chandra Moskowitz.

You can also make eggless salad with tofu—see our Cajun-Style Eggless Salad recipe (page 261). And yes, you can make a batter for frying without eggs. See our Corny Dog recipe (page 309) for a batter that can be used for frying any kind of food.

VEGGIE MEATS

You will find a wide variety of commercial meat substitutes in the frozen and refrigerated section of grocery stores. Look for burgers, hot dogs, sausages, sandwich slices, meatballs, bacon, pepperoni and more—all cruelty-free and better for you than their meaty counterparts. Be sure to check labels, as some contain dairy or eggs. Many vegans swear by a favorite brand of veggie meats. For some it is Gardein (in both freezer and refrigerator section); for others, it is Field Roast or Tofurky, which each make sausages, sandwich slices, and loaves.

SEITAN

Also called wheat meat, seitan is a chewy, meatlike product made from vital wheat gluten, which is a flour made from wheat protein. You can buy prepared seitan or make it (see our seitan recipes, following, and on pages 277 and 314). Look for vital wheat gluten (also called gluten flour), in the baking section of your grocery or natural foods store.

VEGAN SAUSAGE AND VEGAN MEAT (SEITAN)

This recipe comes from Sandy Weiland (page 158), who wanted to develop her own version of vegan meat. Regular vegan meat (seitan) can be made from this recipe by reducing the salt to 1 teaspoon and omitting the smoked paprika, fennel, and cayenne pepper.

▶ **MAKES 12 TO 15 LINKS**

2 cups vital wheat gluten

2 teaspoons salt

1 tablespoon granulated garlic

2 tablespoons onion powder

1 teaspoon dried oregano

3 tablespoons onion flakes

1 teaspoon freshly ground black pepper

1 teaspoon red pepper flakes

1 teaspoon smoked paprika

2 teaspoons fennel seeds (1 teaspoon ground, 1 teaspoon whole)

$\frac{1}{4}$ teaspoon cayenne pepper

$\frac{1}{8}$ teaspoon citric acid

3 tablespoons extra virgin olive oil

$\frac{1}{4}$ cup soy sauce

1. Have ready two 16 × 12-inch pieces of cheesecloth, butcher string, and a steamer pot with a removable basket.

2. Put all the dry ingredients in a large mixing bowl and whisk gently together. Add 1½ cups water, the oil, and soy sauce. Knead the mixture until all the dry ingredients are moistened, then divide in half.

3. Wet the cheesecloth and squeeze out the extra water so the meat won't stick as readily. Spread out the cheesecloth, place one half of the sausage mixture 2 inches from one long end and shape into a roughly 1½ × 12–inch sausage roll. Roll up the sausage in the cheesecloth and tie the ends with string. You should have about 2 inches of cheesecloth hanging off each end of the rolled sausage.

4. Repeat with the other half of the sausage mixture.

5. Put about 3 inches of water in bottom of the steamer pot and insert the steamer. Place the two rolled sausages in the steamer. Cover and bring to a boil. Lower the heat and simmer for 60 minutes, until firm to the touch, checking several times to make sure the water has not boiled away.

6. Let cool and cut the string off the ends of the cheesecloth. Unroll the meat and store covered in the refrigerator for up to 5 days. If making sausages, slice into links. The meat freezes well. The cheesecloth can be machine washed, air dried, and reused.

SOY CURLS

Made by Butler Foods from textured whole soybeans, Soy Curls are a fast and easy way to add meaty texture to sandwiches and casseroles. They need to be rehydrated before cooking. Try them instead of chicken in chicken salad. Or soak them in hot water flavored with tamari and a little bit of liquid smoke, then sauté for a crispy treat that can stand in for bacon in any recipe. Find them at local natural foods stores or online at VeganEssentials.com.

TEXTURED VEGETABLE PROTEIN (TVP®)

This fun soy food is easy to use. Textured vegetable protein comes dry in crumbles that are rehydrated with water or vegetable broth. It absorbs the flavors in any dish in which it's included, but works best as a ground beef substitute in tomato-based dishes such as pasta sauce, Sloppy Joes and chili.

VEGAN "PULLED PORK"

The fruit of the Southeast Asian jackfruit tree has a unique texture that is remarkably similar to shredded pork. Look for young green jackfruit canned in water or brine (not syrup). It's usually available at Asian markets.

▶ **SERVES 2 TO 4**

One 20-ounce can young jackfruit in water or brine
¾ cup vegan BBQ Sauce (see page 277 for our recipe)

1. Drain the jackfruit and chop it roughly. Add the vegan BBQ Sauce and ¼ cup of water. Simmer over low heat for 30 minutes, or cook on low in a slow cooker for several hours to allow the seasonings to work their way into the jackfruit. (You could also sauté an onion, a couple of jalapeño peppers, and a few garlic cloves and add to the jackfruit.)

VARIATION: Jackfruit can also be used in lettuce wraps (see Fast Festive Foods, page 269). For this, omit the barbecue sauce and cook it for 30 minutes in 1 cup of vegetable broth seasoned with 1 teaspoon of minced fresh ginger and 1 tablespoon of hoisin sauce.

VEGAN BACON

Many people use Fakin' Bacon (made from tempeh), or Smart Bacon (made from soy), or Soy Curls (see page 232) as bacon substitutes. You'll even find vegan versions of Canadian bacon.

VEGAN TUNA FISH

For tuna-fish sandwiches you can use mashed chickpeas or tempeh (a cake of fermented soybeans that has a tender and chewy texture and a savory flavor sometimes described as "yeasty" or "mushroom-like"). There are almost as many versions of "mock-tuna salad" in the world as there are vegans. Here is out favorite version.

DOLPHIN- AND TUNA-FRIENDLY MOCK-TUNA SALAD

This recipe makes a wonderful sandwich spread, or it can be stuffed into tomatoes to serve for a fancy luncheon. Kelp granules is the secret ingredient here. They give this salad a little bit of tunalike flavor. (Look for kelp granules in the spice section of natural foods markets or order them from veganessentials.com.) This recipe makes a wonderful sandwich spread, or it can be stuffed into tomatoes to serve for a fancy luncheon.

▶ MAKES 4 CUPS (ENOUGH FOR 4 SANDWICHES)

Two 15-ounce cans chickpeas, drained and rinsed, or 3 cups
    cooked chickpeas
½ cup coarsely chopped onion
½ cup coarsely chopped celery
¼ cup vegan mayonnaise, or to taste
1 tablespoon fresh lemon juice
1 teaspoon kelp granules, or to taste

1. Place the chickpeas in a bowl and coarsely mash them with a potato masher or a pastry blender. The chickpeas should be a little on the chunky side. Add the remaining ingredients and mix everything thoroughly.

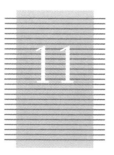

11

RECIPES FOR EVERYDAY
AND FESTIVE EATING

RECIPES IN THIS CHAPTER

SOUPS, STEWS, AND CHILIS

Carrot Coconut Soup

Portuguese Kale Soup

Red Lentil Soup with
Curry

Fast, Filling Chili

SANDWICHES AND SANDWICH SPREADS

Mushroom Pâté

Red Pepper and White Bean Spread
with Cashews

BBQ "Beef" Sandwiches with
Beef-Style Seitan

Groovin' Reuben

VEGETABLE DISHES

Roasted Veggies and Tofu

Spicy Collards with
Ginger

Kale with Cinnamon

Greens and Mushrooms

Sweet and Sour Red Cabbage

Mashed Potatoes and Gravy

White Bean Gravy with Ginger
and Cinnamon

Yum Puk Good (Thai-Style
Asparagus)

Tsimmis (Holiday Baked Yam
Casserole)

SPICE MIXES, BEANS, AND GRAINS

Chinese Five-Spice Seasoning

Creole Seasoning

Herbes de Provence

Greek Seasonings

Mild Indian Curry Seasoning

Italian Seasoning

Jamaican Heat Wave Spice

Heat Wave Beans

Almond-Miso Sauce

Festive Quinoa

Christina's Black-Bean Burgers
with Mango BBQ Sauce

Beans and Greens

MAIN-COURSE MEALS

"Chicken" Piccata

Helen R. Moy's Mac and Cheese

Lasagna

Tempeh and Vegetables with
Indonesian Peanut Sauce

Mediterranean Chickpeas

Sweet and Spicy Baked Tofu

Tracy's Quick Enchiladas

Corny Dogs with a Vegan Frying
Batter

Neatloaf

Turkey's Favorite Bread Dressing

Shirley's Moussaka

Stuffed Seitan Roast

DESSERTS

Zucchini Bread

Mom's Vegan Cinnamon Rolls

Marzipan and Strawberries Dipped
in Chocolate

Hummingbird Cake

Texas Chocolate Sheet Cake

Banana Cake

OUR VEGAN LIVES

Foods We Like to Prepare

Patti: One of my favorite meals is a baked potato or sweet potato topped with sautéed onions and mushrooms. I sauté the chopped onion in ¼ cup of vegetable broth until it is translucent. Then I add sliced mushrooms and cook them until they brown. Sometimes I add a little more broth, if needed, but usually I cook them just until the liquid is absorbed.

Another favorite is a bowl of grains (brown rice or quinoa usually) topped with some avocado, broccoli, toasted sesame seeds, and a very little bit of ume plum vinegar.

And my favorite breakfast is a bowl of oatmeal with fruit, flaxseeds, and soy milk or a huge green smoothie with flaxseeds and whatever greens and fruit are on hand.

I live in a townhouse without great light and very little space for growing vegetables. A few summers back, after three years on a waiting list, I finally got a plot in the community garden behind my local library. Now, with the help of my expert gardener friend Peter Greene, I grow kale, collards, tomatoes, basil, cukes, peas, carrots, potatoes, and flowers. What a joy to be able to create meals and decorate the table straight from the earth! If the me from thirty years ago was told I would be a vegan and growing some of my own food, she'd have laughed and not believed it. But here I am!

Carol: In the summer, I love to make my own version of gazpacho, by starting with a quarter of a bunch of kale and about a cup of basil leaves. I blend them together with a 32-ounce can of roasted tomatoes, ½ cup of vegetable stock, and ¼ cup of red wine vinegar. Then I pulse a seeded cucumber, one green or red pepper, and one sweet onion. I adjust the seasonings and add a little hot pepper sauce, such as Tabasco, and refrigerate for several hours. At serving time, I'll make some garlic and oregano croutons. This is practically a dinner in a bowl, so I don't serve a main dish, but often several salads—say, a tofu salad (an egg salad recipe that is replaced by tofu) or tempeh salad.

When it is cooler, I want to roast oyster mushrooms and serve them over quinoa with some roasted bok choy and baked tofu. On days that I feel the urge to cook something elaborate, I might be found trying out my own recipe for chiles rellenos or stuffed seitan.

When I cook a recipe from a book, I always mark what day I prepared it and make comments. (Too much mustard; not enough liquid, etc.)

Every year for Thanksgiving and Christmas, I make a menu list a few days ahead of time, and figure out what day I should make what dish. For many years I made a mushroom cobbler and walnut "Cheddar" balls (those recipes are in Living Among Meat Eaters). But our current favorite is the Stuffed Seitan Roast (page 314), and it is fun to prepare it in advance and freeze it till it is needed

Living in Dallas, I have the opportunity to have vegan Vietnamese pho for a lunch meeting, or a vegan BBQ sandwich at the local vegan diner. At home, I like to combine a variety of veggies and roast them. When Patti mentioned a "bacon," lettuce, and tomato sandwich that got me thinking of other sandwiches I hadn't tried in a long time.

I think I am still so tickled about vegan food, that I continually enjoy both doing something new and preparing the tried and true.

Ginny: I love good food, but I often don't have time to cook. So I gravitate toward easily prepared basics—baked sweet potatoes, sautéed tofu, quinoa, braised greens, for example—topped with some kind of fabulous sauce.

I almost always have a jar of homemade peanut sauce and one of tofu-cashew sauce in the fridge. I use the peanut sauce that's on page 304 in this book. For the tofu cashew sauce, I blend together until smooth (in a food processor or blender) one 12-ounce package of soft silken tofu, a handful of raw cashews, and 2 tablespoons each of nutritional yeast, sesame tahini, and fresh lemon juice, plus a tablespoon of Dijon mustard. I might toss a clove of garlic in, too. And enough water to make it "saucy." It is wonderful over grains, any steamed vegetable, or baked white or sweet potatoes.

I also make bean burritos with black beans and onions, topped with a little vegan cheese and served with chunks of avocado and very spicy salsa. And I like Old World soups—lentil, vegetable, or pasta and bean soups. My favorite meal is one that I had in Taormina, Italy, on the island of Sicily, and that is easily created at home: chickpeas baked with tomatoes, garlic, oregano, and olive oil, served with a salad of lettuce and chicory, some freshly baked crusty bread, and a glass (or two) of Chianti.

I eat at least one huge (in a mixing bowl!) salad every day of mixed greens, beans, walnuts, shredded cabbage, and shredded carrots, tossed with extra virgin olive oil and balsamic vinegar.

And, of course, when time is short, I'm happy to reach for a microwaved veggie burger on a whole wheat bun with ketchup and pickles, plus prewashed salad from a bag. My cooking style varies from day to day but there are plenty of vegan menu ideas to suit my mood and schedule.

SHORTCUTS IN THE KITCHEN

WHEN YOUR TIME IS limited, or your food supply is lacking, you can easily use these shortcuts and convenience foods in many recipes.

▶ Chopped garlic, packed in water, in a jar. Or, frozen, chopped garlic. (The frozen form is available at Trader Joe's, and it comes packaged in little trays.)

▶ Although fresh lemon juice may taste more alive than the bottled or frozen variety, the difference in their flavors is subtle, so substituting with these versions is well worth doing if it helps you in making the dish.

▶ Here's another shortcut for lemons. When you're squeezing a lemon for its juice, using the following method will save you the time and effort of having to search for and retrieve the seeds that often pop out and land right in whatever you may be making. Hold and squeeze the half lemon with its flat, exposed, open half facing upward. This will allow all the liquid to flow over and out and the seeds to rise to the top where you can easily scrape them off.

▶ When adding fresh ginger or citrus peel, use a Microplane grater, which is a long, narrow, fine grater. Hold or rest the grater across the diameter of any bowl or pot and grate the ginger or peel directly into whatever you are preparing.

▶ When preparing any grain, during the last 3 to 5 minutes of cooking, use the same pot to add and steam any veggies.

BREAKFAST

Many of us, vegan or not, often eat the same thing for breakfast day after day. Perhaps we are more ambitious on weekends or more creative when guests are visiting, but for the most part, we like our mornings to be routine.

Many frequently eaten breakfasts are already vegan, although you may not have thought of yours as such. Oatmeal, for one, can be prepared quickly, and with berries or other fruit and cinnamon it can be one of the healthiest and tastiest ways to start your day (see pages 242 and 243 for two oatmeal variations). Oatmeal aside, any whole grain can be soaked overnight and heated in the morning. Many people fill a slow cooker at night and enjoy a ready-made breakfast in the morning. And toast with peanut or almond butter is a great breakfast, too. When you're in a hurry, leftovers from dinner can be reheated as breakfast.

In many countries, breakfast does not look all that different from lunch and dinner. In Eastern Europe, vegetable salads, especially slaws, are often a major part of breakfast. The classic vegetarian English breakfast is baked beans on toast. Mash the beans (check that they are vegan) with a fork, and top with fresh tomatoes and sautéed mushrooms.

FRUIT SMOOTHIES

Fruit smoothies are a favorite way to create a fast meal that is packed with nutrients and antioxidants. Use any of your favorite fruits: strawberries, blueberries, grapes, mangoes, peaches, and papaya are all good choices. If you like them, bananas, especially when frozen, lend creaminess to any smoothie. You can also get that creamy essence by using silken tofu. In recent years, green smoothies have become even more popular. They are simply fruit smoothies with the addition of green leafy vegetables (kale, spinach, chard, beet greens).

This recipe begins as a fruit smoothie. Add the greens and it becomes a green smoothie. People like to have these alone or with other foods for breakfast, or as a nutritious substitute for any meal at any time. See the additional notes following this recipe.

▶ **MAKES FOUR 6-OUNCE SERVINGS**

1 banana, frozen or fresh
About 1 cup, or more, any juicy fruit, fresh or frozen (except melon), cut into blender-ready size pieces (be sure to remove any pits, cores, and produce stickers)
About 2 cups water or soy, rice, almond, or hemp milk
2 tablespoons ground flaxseeds, optional
2 to 3 or more cups green leafy vegetables, washed and with any thick stems removed
¼ teaspoon or more ground cinnamon, to taste, optional

1. Combine all the ingredients in a blender until smooth, and serve.

NOTES: One favorite combination includes frozen mango, a banana, and plain or vanilla-flavored soy milk. For the greens, any will do. Spinach has the mildest flavor of all, and even young children love this made with it. Mustard greens and arugula have a strong, sharp flavor; use them frugally and mix with a milder green. Or try to include chard, kale, collard, bok choy, parsley, and beet greens.

The mango flavor overtakes the spinach, so, except for the bright green color, no one would guess that the smoothie contains spinach. After you try a spinach smoothie, you can experiment by gradually adding a few leaves of other greens, to see whether you like their flavor. Vary the amounts of fruits and greens and their ratio to liquid until you reach the thickness and flavor you prefer.

Patti uses seven to ten grapes for sweetening, half an orange, an apple, and sometimes a few berries or a peach or pear. If you add blueberries, the green smoothie will become more brown than green, so, if you want the smoothie to remain green, you might consider skipping the blueberries. Strawberries won't change the color much.

VARIATIONS: Here are more combinations to play with, but don't limit yourself to these. Create your own!

- banana, apple (cored), pear (cored), ground cinnamon, collard leaves (stems removed), and water
- banana, peach (pitted), strawberries, kale leaves (stems removed), and soy milk
- banana, grapes, orange, spinach, arugula, and water.

REFRIGERATOR OATMEAL

While there are many variations, the essence of this recipe consists of rolled oats (not instant oats) and requires soaking them overnight. Uncooked oats provide starch that resists digestion by the small intestine, and passes through to the large intestine, where it functions to help prevent chronic disease. This is Carol's breakfast of choice, and it's so delicious her houseguests often ask to take some of the dry mix home. When preparing the dry mix, she always quadruples the recipe. The key is to remember, every night, to have your breakfast make itself in the refrigerator overnight.

▶ **SERVES 6**

2 cups large rolled oats (not instant oats)
½ cup dried fruit (chopped dates, whole raisins, or dried blueberries)
½ cup walnuts
½ cup almonds
½ cup hemp seeds
½ cup chia seeds
½ cup pumpkin seeds
2 to 4 tablespoons ground cinnamon
Plant-based milk of your choice or half milk and half soy or
    almond yogurt
Blueberries, peaches, bananas, or other fruit, optional

1. Combine the oats, dried fruit, nuts, seeds, and cinnamon and store in a dry, sealed container.

2. Before going to bed, combine ½ cup of the oat mixture with 1 cup of your plant-based milk of choice and refrigerate it. In the morning, add fresh fruit, if desired, to the soaked oat mixture.

UP FROM OATMEAL

The soluble fiber content of oats makes them a powerful food for helping to reduce blood cholesterol. This recipe derives its benefits from two heart-healthy grains—oats and hulled barley (hulled barley is less processed than pearl barley). It comes from our friend, registered dietitian Brenda Davis, who says the recipe has evolved over the years. She says she often replaces part of the oats or barley with other grains, such as Kamut or spelt (which are available in the natural foods section of many grocery stores), and we present this version of the recipe here. Make this hearty breakfast even more nutritious by adding hemp seeds or pumpkin seeds. This recipe makes a large quantity—you'll have enough to last the week!

▶ SERVES 12

½ cup Kamut berries
½ cup spelt berries
½ cup hulled barley
½ cup oat groats
2 to 3 cinnamon sticks, optional
Sweetener of choice, optional, for serving
Chopped nuts or seeds, optional, for serving
Soy or almond milk, optional, for serving
Chopped fruit or berries, optional, for serving

Slow-cooker instructions:
1. Place 8 cups of water, the grains, and the cinnamon sticks in a slow cooker and cook overnight on low.

Stovetop instructions:
1. Bring 8 cups of water to a boil in a large saucepan and add the grains and cinnamon sticks. Lower the heat to a simmer. Cover and let cook until soft (about 90 minutes).

2. Whether slow-cooked or prepared on the stovetop, remove the cinnamon sticks before serving, then, if desired, add your favorite sweeteners, chopped nuts or seeds, soy or almond milk, and chopped fruit or berries.

APPLE BLUEBERRY PANCAKES

Pancakes are so easy to make, but somehow they always feel like a treat. These are good for breakfast or dessert.

▶ MAKES 12 MEDIUM PANCAKES

½ cup all-purpose flour

½ cup whole wheat pastry flour

1 tablespoon organic sugar (see box on page 228)

2 tablespoons baking powder

⅛ teaspoon salt

1 cup plain soy milk

2 tablespoons vegetable oil

½ cup cored and coarsely chopped apple

½ cup fresh or frozen blueberries

Vegan margarine, for cooking

Warm pure maple syrup, for serving

1. Combine the flours, sugar, baking powder, and salt in a bowl. Add the soy milk and vegetable oil and mix just enough to combine. Then fold in the apple and blueberries.

2. Melt the margarine in a large skillet over medium heat. Spoon the pancake batter into the pan—use about ¼ cup of batter per pancake. Let the pancakes cook until the edges begin to bubble. Then flip the pancakes and cook them until they're browned. Repeat to make more pancakes. Serve them with warm maple syrup.

SCRAMBLED TOFU

If you're accustomed to eating eggs for breakfast, you may be surprised to find how appealing this tofu-based alternative is. Vary the scramble in any way you like—see the variations for suggestions. The turmeric gives the tofu an egglike color.

▶ SERVES 4

1 tablespoon extra virgin olive oil

3 garlic cloves, minced

8 to 10 medium mushrooms, sliced

½ cup grated carrot

½ cup sliced scallions, white and light green parts only

1 pound firm tofu, crumbled or cubed

3 tablespoons nutritional yeast

¼ teaspoon ground turmeric

1 tablespoon soy sauce

1 cup spinach leaves

1. Heat the oil in a large skillet over medium-high heat, then sauté the garlic and mushrooms until golden on one side. As you flip the garlic and mushrooms over, add the carrot and scallions. Sauté them together for about 2 minutes.

2. Add the tofu, nutritional yeast, turmeric, and soy sauce. Stir them all together and cook for about 5 minutes.

3. Add the spinach, and let it cook for about 1 minute, or just until it becomes slightly wilted but still holds its shape.

VARIATIONS

- Use oyster or shiitake mushrooms instead of the regular mushrooms.
- Add black olives and sun-dried tomatoes.
- Buy seasoned vegan burgers and substitute for the tofu (Southwest flavor works well). Crumble them into a skillet, heat, and serve with or without added mushrooms.
- Substitute ½ cup of kale torn from the stem for the spinach.
- Add steamed or roasted asparagus.
- While sautéing the veggies, add 1 diced red pepper and 1 cup cooked potato; when you remove the scramble from the heat, add ½ cup salsa and 1 avocado.

VEGANIZING BRUNCH

AS A NEW VEGAN, you may feel a little stymied by the idea of vegan brunch. In fact, the possibilities are fun and easy. Mix and match the recipes in this book with a few store-bought items to keep things manageable. Here are some ideas:

- ▶ pancakes (see recipe, pages 244)
- ▶ Scrambled Tofu (page 245), or scramble some cubed tempeh with peppers and greens
- ▶ a large fruit salad
- ▶ Zucchini Bread (page 317)
- ▶ BLTs (see box on page 276)
- ▶ potatoes roasted with rosemary and garlic
- ▶ vegan sausages (pick them up at your local grocery store or use the recipe on page 231)
- ▶ Cinnamon Rolls (page 318)
- ▶ bagels and vegan cream cheese
- ▶ quesadillas (tortillas usually stuffed with cheese)—substitute a commercial-brand vegan cheese that melts (e.g., Daiya or Teese)
- ▶ Hot Artichoke Dip (page 252)

When you serve any of your new veganized meals, there is no need to call attention to their vegan nature. Let your friends, family, guests, and co-workers simply enjoy the food. Remember our advice: People are perfectly happy eating vegan food as long as they don't know that is what they are doing. As all these tips and suggestions in this chapter show, brunch is a great time to veganize!

APPETIZERS AND DIPS

RAE SIKORA'S CROCK CHEESE

Rae, an advocate, activist, and educator concerning animals, human rights, and the environment, prepared this appetizer when Carol was visiting her, and it has become a staple for Carol to serve to guests. It's quick to prepare, and it's addictive!

▶ **SERVES 6 TO 8**

> 1 cup raw, organic cashews
> 4 ounces red pimientos (come in 4-ounce jars)
> ½ cup fresh lemon juice
> 6 tablespoons nutritional yeast
> 1 teaspoon salt, or to taste
> 1 teaspoon onion powder
> ½ teaspoon garlic powder

1. Process the cashews in a food processor or a blender, until powdery. Add the remaining ingredients and process together until very smooth. Chill. Serve with crackers.
2. If you want a spreadable cheese, double the amount of cashews.

TOFU CHEESE LOG

Use this variation on Tofu Ricotta (page 223) to make a fancy cheese log for a party. Guests enjoy both the flavor and the presentation. They won't even know that it's full of calcium and protein.

▶ **MAKES ONE CHEESE LOG THAT SERVES 4 TO 6**

Cheese:
> 2 garlic cloves, peeled

1 pound firm or extra-firm tofu, pressed

1 teaspoon fresh lemon juice

2 teaspoons extra virgin olive oil

½ teaspoon salt

2 tablespoons white miso

1 tablespoon finely chopped fresh rosemary

Crust:

2 to 3 tablespoons chopped fresh basil

2 garlic cloves, minced

⅓ cup pine nuts or chopped walnuts

1. Make the cheese: Mince the garlic in a food processor. Add the remaining cheese ingredients and process until smooth.

2. Place the cheese mixture on a large piece of plastic wrap. Rock the mixture back and forth, using the plastic wrap to guide it, until it forms a loglike shape. Wrap securely in the plastic and refrigerate for at least 1 hour. You can also prepare this the day before and leave it in the refrigerator overnight.

3. Prepare the crust: Stir together the basil, garlic, and pine nuts.

4. Preheat the oven to 375°F. Remove the tofu roll from the refrigerator. Unwrap the roll but leave it on the plastic. Sprinkle the nut mixture onto the plastic wrap, and roll the tofu over the nut mixture until the tofu is evenly covered.

5. Remove the plastic wrap and place the log on a baking sheet. Bake for 25 minutes.

6. Serve with your favorite bread or crackers.

BASIC HUMMUS

Hummus is a staple for many vegans. Use it as a spread on bread, as a dip, or as a filling in red peppers, pita (pocket bread), or tomatoes. Or use it as a salad dressing, thinned with water, a little olive oil, or additional lemon juice. It's a protein-packed recipe that also delivers a little bit of calcium from the chickpeas and sesame tahini.

▶ **SERVES 6**

One 15-ounce can chickpeas, drained and rinsed
2 tablespoons sesame tahini, or more to taste
3 tablespoons fresh lemon juice, or more to taste
1 garlic clove, minced
⅛ to ¼ teaspoon salt, or to taste

1. Combine all the ingredients in a food processor. Process until they form a smooth paste, adding water, as needed, to thin. Use a spatula to scrape any remaining paste from the sides of the processor bowl. Transfer to a small bowl to serve either at room temperature or chilled, with pita wedges, crackers, or carrots, celery, and broccoli.

VARIATIONS

- For a festive, speckled look, add ¼ cup of chopped fresh parsley to the ingredients while they're in the processor.
- Add one roasted or fresh red pepper, chopped, to the processor. This will give the hummus an appealing red tint.
- Add 2 tablespoons of chopped, pitted black olives to the processor. (Eliminate the salt before adding the olives and taste before deciding to add any.)
- When the hummus is ready, top it with a sprinkle of toasted pine nuts.

CASHEW HERB PÂTÉ

Save money by purchasing nuts in bulk. You'll find a variety of nuts sold in bulk bins in most supermarkets. And, if you can find cashew pieces instead of whole cashews, they cost even less. Soaking the nuts and seeds for an hour or more before preparing this pâté will give it a creamier texture.

▶ **SERVES 6**

1 cup unsalted, raw cashews, soaked in water for an hour or more
½ cup sunflower seeds, soaked in water for an hour or more
Several sprinkles of hot pepper sauce, such as Tabasco (for mild, 1 to
    4 drops; for strong, 5 to10 drops; for very strong, 10-plus drops)
Juice of 1 or 2 lemons
1 teaspoon grated fresh ginger
2 tablespoons chopped fresh parsley
Salt, to taste

1. Drain the nuts and seeds, then combine all the ingredients in a food processor. Process for several minutes, until a thick paste is formed. Transfer to a small bowl and serve with crudités or crackers.

BLACK BEAN DIP

This sweet and spicy dip is wonderful with pita wedges or whole-grain crackers. Making it the day before will allow the flavors plenty of time to develop.

▶ **SERVES 4 TO 6**

1 tablespoon extra virgin olive oil
½ cup finely chopped onion
1 cup cooked black beans, well drained
½ teaspoon garlic powder
½ teaspoon celery powder
⅛ teaspoon freshly ground black pepper
2 tablespoons vegan Worcestershire sauce
⅛ teaspoon hot pepper sauce, such as Tabasco
1 tablespoon sugar

1. Heat the oil in a small skillet over medium heat and sauté the onion until tender. Transfer the onion and remaining ingredients to

a food processor. Process together until smooth. Adjust the seasonings to taste. Transfer to a serving bowl. If not serving immediately, refrigerate; bring the dip to room temperature before serving.

HOT ARTICHOKE DIP

This buffet favorite is traditionally packed with dairy products but is every bit as good with some easy vegan tweaks.

▶ **SERVES 12 AS AN APPETIZER**

One 14-ounce can artichoke hearts, drained and chopped
2 cups vegan mayonnaise (see page 228)
One 8-ounce package vegan cream cheese, softened
1 cup shredded vegan mozzarella cheese, such as Daiya brand
½ cup grated vegan Parmesan, such as Go Veggie! brand, or try
    our recipe (page 224)
Dash of vegan Worcestershire sauce
Salt and freshly ground black pepper

1. Preheat the oven to 350°F.
2. Combine all the ingredients in a large bowl. Mix together and transfer to an 8-inch baking dish, pie plate, or shallow gratin dish. Bake for 25 to 30 minutes, until the top is golden brown and the dip is bubbling.
3. Serve hot with crackers or crostini.

VARIATIONS: There are so many variations on the traditional version of this recipe that you should feel free to adjust the ingredients to suit your taste. You might decide that using 2 cups of vegan mayo plus cream cheese is just too rich. Cut back on the mayo and substitute silken tofu for some (or all) of it, and replace some of the cheese with nutritional yeast for a dip that is a little bit lower in calories. The recipe may need a little nudging if you do this—perhaps the addition of 1 tablespoon of Dijon mustard and 1 tablespoon of fresh lemon juice.

NACHO SAUCE

Everybody loves nachos. Carol made this recipe for a youth group that visited her, and both the children and the accompanying adults reported that they heartily enjoyed the dish.

▶ **SERVES 4 TO 8**

½ cup nutritional yeast
½ cup all-purpose flour
1 teaspoon salt
½ teaspoon garlic powder
4 tablespoons (½ stick) vegan margarine
One 10-ounce can Ro*Tel tomatoes, or 1 small jar mild picante
sauce

1. Mix the dry ingredients together in a saucepan, then add 2 cups of water and cook over medium heat, whisking, until the mixture thickens and bubbles. Remove from the heat and add the margarine.
2. Coarsely chop the tomatoes and add them to the sauce. Serve the sauce warm, with vegan chips.

NOTE: Ro*Tel tomatoes were developed in Texas, in the 1940s, and the brand is still widely available and popular today. Ro*Tel packages, among other products, a combination of canned tomatoes, chiles, and spices that is available in mild or hot form. (But, just remember, hot is hot!) Its popularity spread throughout the South and it became a staple ingredient in *queso* recipes

CRANBERRY FIG RELISH

This crowd-pleaser is a must on Thanksgiving, but don't hesitate to use it at any time of year (although outside of autumn, when fresh cranberries are widely available, you will probably have to use frozen cranberries). Serve it with baked sweet potatoes or Neatloaf (page 310).

▶ **MAKES 5 CUPS**

4 cups fresh or frozen cranberries (see note)
1 cup dried figs, stems removed
2 tablespoons snipped and chopped fresh mint leaves
1 cup orange marmalade
2 tablespoons balsamic vinegar

1. Use a food processor to coarsely chop the cranberries and figs. Transfer to a bowl, and add the mint.

2. Stir together the marmalade and balsamic vinegar. Add to the cranberry and fig mixture and stir well.

3. Cover and refrigerate the relish for a minimum of 2 hours or up to 1 week. Or freeze it for up to 6 months; thaw it in a refrigerator overnight before serving.

NOTE: If the cranberries are frozen, measure them while they're still frozen. Then let them sit at room temperature for about 15 minutes, to thaw slightly before processing.

SALADS AND DRESSINGS

Sometimes the only difference between a snack and a meal is the addition of a salad. And salads can sometimes be meals all by themselves. We've separated out main-dish salads from those presented in this section; those more substantial salads begin on page 261.

WALNUT VINAIGRETTE

Skip bottled dressings from the store; it's so easy to make your own. This one will take you about two minutes to make, and it uses heart-healthy olive oil along with walnut oil, which provides omega-3 fats. You can use this to dress any salad, and it also makes a lovely dressing for warm, roasted root vegetables, such as beets, potatoes, or sweet potatoes. This makes enough for about four servings of salad, so feel free to double, triple, or even quadruple the recipe. The vinaigrette will keep for a week or so refrigerated in a tightly covered jar.

▶ **MAKES ABOUT ¼ CUP**

1 tablespoon sherry or red wine vinegar
1 teaspoon balsamic vinegar
¼ teaspoon salt
1 tablespoon walnut oil
3 tablespoons extra virgin olive oil

1. Place all the ingredients in a jar and shake to combine.

YOGURT-TAHINI DRESSING

This Mediterranean-inspired dressing pairs well with fresh greens, steamed vegetables, or a pita pocket stuffed with falafel and chopped vegetables.

▶ **MAKES ABOUT 2 CUPS**

1 garlic clove, crushed
½ cup sesame tahini
½ cup fresh lemon juice
½ cup plain soy or almond yogurt
1 tablespoon extra virgin olive oil

1. Place all ingredients and ¼ cup of water in a blender or food processor and blend until smooth. Add more water, if needed. The flavors will intensify during refrigeration, so we recommend preparing the dressing several hours ahead of time. However, Patti seldom waits when a recipe calls for waiting. She may be missing out on a better blend of flavors, but nothing seems to be lost by her impatience.

BUILD A SALAD

SALADS CAN BE AS simple as you want—prewashed lettuce or spinach topped with cherry tomatoes is a perfectly good side salad or snack. But in just a few minutes it's easy to build a salad that makes a filling and satisfying meal. You probably have a few items in your refrigerator or pantry right now that can go in a salad: canned beans, nuts, toasted seeds, chopped apples, shredded cabbage, soy "bacon" bits, chunks of baked tofu, sun-dried tomatoes, diced figs, or shredded vegan cheese. Dress your creation with a fast dressing of seasoned rice vinegar, oil and vinegar, or a bottled dressing.

Here are the basic building blocks to a delicious salad; vary which foods you select from each section and you can have a different salad every day of the month!

Greens: red leaf, green leaf, butter, Boston, romaine lettuce. But also think beyond lettuce by using kale, chard, or spinach—all good sources of vitamin A. Why not try bok choy or Chinese cabbage? Massaged Kale Salad (page 260) is a great base for any type of salad.

Raw veggies: shredded or diced carrots, sliced celery, sliced fennel, peppers, tomatoes, broccoli, cauliflower, cabbage, shredded beets, mushrooms, jicama, cucumber, zucchini, summer squash, onions, radishes, scallions (white and green parts), avocado, snow peas, shelled fresh peas

Cooked veggies: cubed baked squash (remove the seeds, if winter squash), cubed baked sweet potatoes, steamed green beans, sliced roasted beets, steamed sugar snap peas

Nuts and seeds: toasted walnuts, cashews, almonds, filberts, hazelnuts, Brazil nuts, sesame seeds, sunflower seeds, pumpkin seeds, pine nuts

Beans: chickpeas, kidney beans, pinto beans, cannellini beans, black beans, Anasazi beans, edamame

Herbs: chopped fresh parsley, cilantro, basil, chives, dill, summer savory, mint, marjoram, oregano, tarragon, thyme, watercress

Fruit: blueberries, strawberries, raspberries, cherries, apples, dried or fresh figs

Store-bought: Sun-dried tomatoes, baked tofu, olives, capers, artichoke hearts, veggie bacon or bacon bits, croutons, cooked and crumbled veggie burger

A FEW OF OUR FAVORITE COMBINATIONS

▶ Chickpeas, sliced fennel, diced tomatoes, olives, red onion, and parsley on a bed of greens

▶ Tomatoes, cannellini beans, green pepper, and fresh basil, on a bed of greens

▶ Romaine lettuce, tomato, red bell pepper, avocado, and sunflower seeds

▶ Spinach plus salad: spinach and kale with mushrooms and croutons

▶ Chopped salad: celery, carrots, red onion, peppers, and romaine topped with baked tofu (toss the tofu in some vegan BBQ Sauce [see recipe page 277] for a delicious variation).

VERY BENEVOLENT CAESAR SALAD DRESSING

Miyoko Schinner, author of the wonderful *Artisan Vegan Cheese*, created this delicious healthy version of a Caesar dressing. You can buy almond meal or make your own by grinding almonds in a coffee grinder or food processor. Use more or less garlic and mustard to suit your taste.

▶ SERVES 4

2 tablespoons almond meal

3 garlic cloves, pressed through a garlic press

3 tablespoons Dijon mustard

¼ cup nutritional yeast flakes

2 tablespoons soy sauce
3 tablespoons fresh lemon juice
¼ cup water

1. Combine the almond meal, garlic, mustard, and nutritional yeast to make a paste, then whisk in the remaining ingredients. This will keep for one week in the refrigerator.

CONFETTI SLAW

Shirley Wilkes-Johnson created this refreshing coleslaw recipe. Serve it on sandwiches or as a side with any meal. Don't worry about having exactly the right quantities of shredded cabbage and carrots—this recipe will turn out beautifully even if you have a little more or a little less of both.

▶ **SERVES 6 TO 8**

6 to 8 cups shredded green cabbage
1 cup shredded carrots
1 large, red, organic apple, cored and diced
¼ cup dried cherries or golden raisins, or both
4 scallions, white and green parts, thinly sliced
1 cup vegan mayonnaise
1 tablespoon fresh lemon juice or cider vinegar
2 tablespoons organic sugar (see box on page 228)
1 teaspoon dried tarragon
¼ teaspoon salt

1. Combine the cabbage, carrots, apple, cherries, and scallions in a large salad bowl. Whisk together the vegan mayonnaise, lemon juice, sugar, tarragon, and salt in a smaller bowl.
2. Pour the dressing over the cabbage mixture, and toss. If possible, chill the slaw before serving.

TOMATO AND PEACH SALAD

Tomatoes and peaches are in peak season at exactly the same time in most places. They make a colorful and surprising combination in this light salad, which is perfect for warm days.

▶ SERVES 4

3 ripe tomatoes, cut into wedges
4 ripe peaches, pitted and cut into chunks
¼ small red onion, sliced
½ cup chopped fresh cilantro
Juice of 1 lime or lemon

1. Combine all the ingredients and serve at room temperature.

SWEET POTATO SALAD WITH PECANS

This salad is a favorite at Ginny's Thanksgiving dinner. It's also a great choice when you want something that's a little different for a picnic or potluck.

▶ SERVES 8

4 medium sweet potatoes, peeled and cut into ¾-inch chunks
4 celery stalks, thinly sliced
1 small red bell pepper, seeded and coarsely chopped
1 cup diced pineapple
2 scallions, white and green parts, thinly sliced
¼ cup vegan mayonnaise
2 tablespoons Dijon mustard
½ cup chopped pecans
Salt and freshly ground black pepper

1. Bring a large pot of water to a boil, add the sweet potatoes, and cook until just tender, 10 to 15 minutes. (Watch to be sure they

don't become too soft.) Allow the sweet potatoes to cool to room temperature. Toss with the celery, red bell pepper, pineapple, and scallions in a large bowl.

2. Mix the mayonnaise and mustard together in a small bowl. Fold the dressing into the sweet potato mixture. Chill for at least 1 hour before serving.

3. Before serving, toast the pecans in a skillet, over medium heat, for 2 to 3 minutes, stirring constantly with a wooden spoon or heat-resistant spatula to prevent them from burning. Fold the pecans into the sweet potato salad. Add salt and pepper to taste.

MASSAGED KALE SALAD

If you've poked around vegan sites on the Internet, you've most likely noticed the kale craze. It's not just that kale is nutritious, it's also beautiful, delicious, and versatile. You don't even need to cook it to enjoy it. You can massage kale to make it soft and add it to or use it as a base for any salad. Massaged kale is especially good served over cooked quinoa or brown rice.

▶ **SERVES 4 TO 6**

1 bunch of any kind of kale: red, curly, lacinato (also called dinosaur kale), washed and dried in a salad spinner or with a towel, stems removed, and chopped or torn into bite-size pieces

¼ to ½ teaspoon salt (start with ¼ teaspoon and add more if you feel it is needed to hasten the softening)

Any other salad fixings you like (cucumber, tomato, avocado, red cabbage, bok choy, red or green onion, carrots, red, yellow or green pepper, etc.)

Juice of ½ or 1 lime or lemon or the salad dressing of your choice (see pages 255–258 for salad dressings)

1. Remove the kale leaves from the stems, enjoying the feeling of the leaves in your fingers. Hold the leafy part in one hand and the stem in the other. Pull up the stem toward the leaf and it will stay in your hand while the leafy part pulls right off. This is like a mini massage for the inside of your thumb and forefinger. It is very tactile and most people find stemming kale leaves enjoyable.

2. Sprinkle the salt on the kale and massage it in with your fingers. Don't be afraid to knead vigorously. The longer you massage, the more tender it will be. It will also lose some volume, as when it's cooked. Massage for 1 to 5 minutes, depending on how soft you want the kale to be.

3. In a large bowl, combine the softened kale with the remaining ingredients.

MAIN-DISH SALADS

CAJUN-STYLE EGGLESS SALAD

Texas vegan chef Shirley Wilkes-Johnson created this incredible eggless salad. It can be spooned on sandwiches or crackers, or served stuffed into cooked and chilled jumbo pasta shells. If you have a deviled-egg plate, arrange the shells in the indentations to serve.

▶ **SERVES 4**

1 pound firm or extra-firm tofu, drained, rinsed, and patted dry
2 tablespoons nutritional yeast
½ teaspoon ground turmeric
½ teaspoon curry powder
½ teaspoon salt, or to taste
⅛ teaspoon ground white pepper
¼ cup finely chopped celery

2 scallions, white and light green parts, thinly sliced

2 tablespoons seeded and finely chopped red pepper

2 tablespoons sliced, pimiento-stuffed olives

⅓ cup vegan mayonnaise, or more as desired

2 tablespoons prepared yellow mustard

1 tablespoon cider vinegar

¼ teaspoon hot pepper sauce, such as Tabasco, optional

Paprika

1. Place the tofu in a large bowl and mash with a fork. Add the remaining ingredients, except the paprika, and mix with a fork until it reaches the consistency of egg salad. Sprinkle the paprika over the top.

MINTED BARLEY SALAD

The traditional Mediterranean flavors of this dish are usually teamed up with couscous. We've used barley instead, to increase the soluble fiber content, which helps to lower cholesterol. But you can substitute any grain you may have on hand.

▶ **SERVES 4**

½ cup uncooked pearled barley

2 tablespoons extra virgin olive oil

1 medium carrot, cut into julienne strips

1 medium zucchini, cut into julienne strips

½ teaspoon ground ginger

2 teaspoons dried mint

½ cup sliced almonds

½ cup raisins

3 tablespoons fresh lemon juice

Salt and freshly ground black pepper

1. Bring 1½ cups of water to a boil in a 2-quart saucepan and add the barley. Cover, and lower the heat to simmer. Cook the barley until all the water is absorbed, about 45 minutes.

2. While the barley is cooking, heat the oil in a large skillet. Add the carrot strips, zucchini strips, ginger, and mint and sauté together for 3 to 4 minutes.

3. Place the cooked barley, sautéed vegetables, almonds, and raisins in a large bowl and toss to combine. Drizzle the lemon juice over the mixture and mix thoroughly.

4. Season with salt and pepper to taste.

FLEXIBLE QUINOA SALAD

Quinoa (pronounced KEEN wah) is a seed that cooks like a grain. This colorful salad can be made with any variety of bean or vegetable and just about any dressing (hence this recipe's name). If you don't have quinoa on hand, you can even make it with brown rice. It can be served warm or cold. The simplest dressing is seasoned rice vinegar, available in most groceries and markets.

▶ SERVES 4

1 cup uncooked quinoa, rinsed (see note)
1 red, green, or yellow pepper, seeded and chopped or diced
1 cup fresh or frozen yellow corn
1 cup fresh or frozen peas
3 cups baby spinach, washed and dried
½ to 1 cup finely cut or shredded red cabbage, optional
¼ cup diced, smoked tofu, baked tofu, or black beans, optional
3 tablespoons seasoned rice vinegar
¼ teaspoon ground cumin, optional
Juice of 1 lime or lemon, optional

1. Bring 2 cups of water to a boil and add the quinoa. Lower the heat to simmer and cover. Cook until all water is absorbed, about 15 minutes. If you are using frozen corn or peas, add them to the quinoa during the last 3 minutes of cooking time. In a large serving bowl, combine the quinoa, pepper, corn, peas, spinach, and cabbage and tofu, if using; stir together.

2. Combine the rice vinegar with the cumin and citrus juice (if using). Pour over the quinoa mixture and toss gently to mix.

NOTE: Quinoa has a bitter, naturally occurring coating, saponin, to ward off insects. For years it was recommended that quinoa needed to be rinsed before cooking to dissolve the saponin's bitter flavor. Producers of quinoa now report that the bitterness from the saponin has been removed before it is packaged and sold. However, just as with rice, it is always good to rinse first by placing the quinoa in a fine-mesh strainer and holding it under running water for about 90 seconds before cooking.

APRICOT AND WHITE BEAN SALAD

If you don't have apricots on hand use any dried fruit you like to make this quick, substantial salad. Serve it at room temperature, with warm whole-grain bread. It's perfect for backyard barbecues and picnics.

▶ SERVES 4

Two 15-ounce cans small white beans, drained and rinsed, or
    3 cups home-cooked white beans (see pages 294–295)
½ cup coarsely chopped red onion
½ cup finely chopped dried apricots, soaked in ½ cup warm
    water for 30 minutes and then drained
¼ cup halved Kalamata olives
1 teaspoon dried oregano
½ teaspoon dried tarragon

1 tablespoon dried parsley

2 tablespoons extra virgin olive oil

1 tablespoon red wine vinegar

1 teaspoon Dijon mustard

Salt and freshly ground black pepper

1. Combine the beans, onion, apricots, olives, oregano, tarragon, and parsley in a large bowl and gently mix together.

2. Put the olive oil, vinegar, and mustard in a jar, and shake well to combine. Pour the dressing over the salad and toss the salad to distribute the dressing. Add salt and pepper to taste.

QUINOA-STUFFED AVOCADOS

Avocados are not just for guacamole. They make a lovely—and heart-healthy—bowl for quinoa salad.

▶ **SERVES 4**

¾ cup uncooked quinoa, rinsed (see note on the previous page)

2 teaspoons extra virgin olive oil

1 small red onion, minced

1 medium tomato, diced

1 tablespoon minced fresh parsley

½ teaspoon salt

¼ teaspoon freshly ground black pepper

2 ripe avocados

1 tablespoon fresh lemon juice

4 large leaves butter lettuce

1. Bring 1½ cups of water to a boil in a saucepan and add the quinoa. Lower the heat to a simmer and cover. Cook until all the water is absorbed, about 15 minutes. Set aside.

2. Heat 1 teaspoon of the oil in a skillet over medium heat. Add the onion and cook for 5 minutes, or until soft. Transfer to a bowl.

3. Add the cooked quinoa and the tomato, parsley, salt, and pepper to the onion and toss to combine.

4. Cut the avocados in half and remove their pits. (You can accomplish this quickly by thrusting a sharp knife blade into the pit and carefully twisting the knife.) Remove the pulp with a spoon, while keeping the shells intact. Cut the avocados into small chunks, about ½ inch each, and add to the quinoa mixture. Don't worry if the avocado pieces are uneven or messy.

5. Add the lemon juice and remaining teaspoon of oil and gently toss the mixture together.

6. Spoon the mixture into the halved avocado shells and serve them immediately, on salad plates lined with the lettuce leaves.

SOUTHWESTERN CORN SALAD

This colorful salad from Shirley Wilkes-Johnson is perfect for summer luncheons, and even as a Thanksgiving dish. It's well worth the trouble of all the chopping. Be sure to use avocados that are firm but ripe and not soft and mushy.

▶ **SERVES 8 TO 10**

One 16-ounce package frozen corn, thawed

2 cups quartered cherry tomatoes or seeded and diced tomatoes

One 15-ounce can kidney beans, drained and rinsed

1 cup chopped red onion

1 cup diced peeled carrots

½ each red, green, and orange bell peppers, seeded and diced

½ cup chopped fresh cilantro

½ cup black olives, sliced

2 avocados, peeled, pitted, and cut into ½-inch cubes

1 fresh jalapeño pepper, seeded and diced

2 garlic cloves, minced

1 teaspoon ground cumin

1 teaspoon salt

½ teaspoon coarsely ground black pepper

¼ cup fresh lime juice

Lettuce, for serving

1. Put the corn into a large bowl. Add the tomatoes, beans, red onion, carrots, bell peppers, cilantro, and black olives and gently toss. Add the avocado, jalapeño, garlic, cumin, salt, black pepper, and lime juice. Toss gently again, cover, and refrigerate until you're ready to serve. Serve individual portions in lettuce cups.

Easy Vegan Meals for the Noncook

Vegan meals can be as simple or as elaborate as you like. If you love to cook, we hope that some of the recipes in this book will become favorite standbys. But even those of us who enjoy exploring new recipes sometimes, or often, need to get meals on the table without reading and measuring. Most of the cooking we do—omnivores and vegans alike—is built around familiar food preparation that doesn't require a recipe.

Food preparation gets even easier when you let go of "rules" about what to eat and when. Soup for breakfast? It's standard fare in Japan where miso soup is a favorite morning meal.

The ideas below are for "anytime meals." They serve as breakfast or dinner or a snack. And you don't need to know a thing about cooking to prepare them!

Wrap It Up

Fast snack food or elegant party food: wraps can go either way. They are always easy and can use whatever you have on hand. Wrap food in tortillas, chapatis, collard greens, romaine or iceberg lettuce leaves, or sea vegetables. (Nori rolls or sushi are the quintessential Japanese wrap.)

What goes in a wrap? Anything you like! Hummus is a reliable standby, but you can also use refried beans topped with salsa or avocado, Scrambled Tofu (page 245), beans and grains mixed with a little salad dressing or sauce, guacamole, curried vegetables, or tossed salad. Wraps and stuffed vegetables are among the best ways to use up leftovers, including those from a restaurant. Even a small amount of food turns into a meal when you roll it up in a vegan chapati.

Pinwheels cut from wraps are a favorite, especially with grandkids and other visiting young friends and relatives. Spread a tortilla or thin, soft vegan flatbread with vegan cream cheese. Add sliced olives or roasted red peppers, chopped softened sun-dried tomatoes or whatever you like. Sprinkle with herbs and freshly ground black pepper. Roll it up and then slice into rounds. Arrange on a bed of lettuce for maximum effect.

Pinwheels made from peanut or almond butter and shredded carrots—a fun and healthy lunch or snack—may prove especially popular.

Stuffed Vegetables and Fruit

Think of these as a variation on a wrap. You can stuff any veggie (or fruit) that has a hollow inside, such as celery or bell peppers, or you can scoop out the center of cucumbers or zucchini. Anything that goes into a wrap will work as stuffing for a vegetable. The classic kids' snack, Ants on a Log—celery stuffed with peanut butter and topped with raisins—works just fine for us adults, too.

Create an instant food to share with store-bought hummus and a "cone head" of Belgian endive leaves. Pull the leaves apart, spoon hummus into each leaf and arrange on a platter for a beautiful appetizer. Make it fancier by topping each stuffed leaf with a few capers or sliced olives or red peppers if you like.

Stuffed pears are a healthy and satisfying snack, too. Cut a ripe pear in half lengthwise. Scoop out the center stem and seeds with a melon baller or spoon, and fill the groove with sesame tahini or peanut butter.

Go for Convenience (When You Need It)

Canned beans make meal preparation easy. See 5 Things to Do with Canned Beans on page 88. Use any of your favorite condiments—salsa, mustard, seasoned rice vinegar—to quickly dress up beans. Serve them over any cooked grain or as a salad on a bed of lettuce.

Frozen vegetables are just as good for you as fresh, and are often less expensive and faster to prepare (and are available year-round, a nice option for vegetables that are fresh only seasonally). In a pinch, canned vegetables are fine to include in meals, too. They aren't quite as good for you as frozen or fresh, but eating canned veggies is better than skipping veggies altogether.

Soup from a can or box can provide a great starter for your own "homemade" recipe. Add beans, diced cooked potatoes and veggies, and heat it up for ultimate convenience with your own special touch.

And, of course, the vast and ever-growing selection of veggie meats (see chapter 10) means that a home-prepared dinner can be ready in minutes.

5 Fast Festive Foods

1. Stuffed grape leaves: You'll find these canned or in the refrigerator or deli section of some grocery stores, including Costco. Put in a baking dish, add a little vegetable stock and olive oil; sprinkle with pine nuts and lemon slices. Cover with foil and warm at 350°F for 20 minutes.

2. Nachos and guacamole: Buy premade guacamole and add some pico de gallo and chunks of chopped fresh avocado to it. Serve with vegan corn chips. For Super

Nachos, layer warmed refried beans, salsa, Nacho Sauce (see page 253), shredded lettuce, chopped tomatoes. Serve with tortilla chips.

3. Make iceberg lettuce cups like the ones restaurant chain P. F. Chang's is famous for: Form lettuce cups in small bowls or a muffin tin. Fill with tiny, tiny slices of limes, peanuts, sautéed mushrooms, store-bought smoked tofu, shredded coconut, and grated ginger. Serve with hoisin sauce.

4. Prepare vacuum-packed or frozen gnocchi (many brands are vegan) and serve with tomato sauce or olive oil, garlic, and fresh basil.

5. Grill it up! Marinate portobello mushrooms in a balsamic vinaigrette with a little garlic and Italian or French herbs. Grill and serve in whole-grain burger buns along with sliced onions, tomatoes, and lettuce.

SOUPS, STEWS, AND CHILIS

A warm bowl of soup, stew, or chili is comforting any time and especially welcome on cold winter days.

CARROT COCONUT SOUP

Patti often doubles this recipe, as everyone loves it and it's always devoured (it originally appeared on the website for the George Mateljan Foundation World's Healthiest Foods, whfoods.org).

▶ SERVES 4

1 large onion, chopped

3 cups vegan vegetable stock or broth

2 tablespoons sliced fresh ginger, or 1 teaspoon dried

4 garlic cloves, chopped

1 teaspoon curry powder

2 cups sliced carrot

1 cup cubed peeled sweet potato (small cubes)

5 ounces canned coconut milk

Salt and freshly ground black pepper

1. Sauté the onion in ¼ cup of the vegetable stock in a medium-size soup pot for about 5 minutes, stirring often.

2. Add the fresh ginger and garlic and continue to sauté for another minute. Add the curry powder. If you are not using fresh ginger, this is the time to add the dried ginger.

3. Add remaining stock, carrot, and sweet potato and simmer over medium-high heat until the vegetables are tender, about 15 minutes.

4. Transfer the stock and vegetables to a blender. Add coconut milk by blending it in batches, making sure the blender is never more than half full. When the contents of the blender are hot and the blender is more than half full, the ingredients can easily erupt and inflict burns. (Alternatively, if you have cut up the veggies in small enough pieces, you can use an immersion blender.)

5. Add salt and pepper to taste. Return the blended ingredients to the soup pot and reheat.

PORTUGUESE KALE SOUP

We like to make this with Tofurky brand Apple and Sage Sausage, but any commercial vegan sausage will work in this healthy version of the national soup of Portugal. Serve with a loaf of crusty bread for a hearty and satisfying meal.

▶ **SERVES 8**

¼ cup extra virgin olive oil

1 large yellow onion, coarsely chopped

3 garlic cloves, minced

2 pounds small white or red potatoes, halved and
    thinly sliced

1 pound fresh kale

8 ounces vegan sausage, coarsely chopped

2 quarts vegan vegetable stock or broth

Salt and freshly ground black pepper

1. Wash the kale and tear it into bite-size pieces, discarding the stems. Set it aside.

2. Heat the olive oil in a large, heavy pot over medium heat. Add the onion and sauté until tender. Add the garlic and potatoes and stir to coat well with the oil. Cook for another 3 minutes.

3. Add the kale, sausage, vegetable broth, salt, and pepper to the pot. Stir to combine the ingredients. Bring to a boil and then reduce the heat to simmer. Cover the pot and simmer until the potatoes are tender, about 20 minutes.

RED LENTIL SOUP WITH CURRY

Lentils and barley both provide plenty of soluble fiber, the kind that lowers blood cholesterol. You can make this with any type of lentils you like, but red lentils—which actually turn yellow as they cook—produce a soup with a pureed quality. You can also use a little bit less water to make a thicker soup that can stand in for a sauce over potatoes or vegetables.

▶ SERVES 8

1 onion, chopped

2 carrots, peeled and diced

2 to 3 or more garlic cloves, minced

8 cups vegan vegetable stock or broth or water

2 cups red lentils

⅓ cup pearled barley

1 tablespoon curry powder, or to taste

1 teaspoon grated fresh ginger

Pinch of freshly grated nutmeg

Salt and freshly ground pepper

Handful of raw or steamed chopped greens,
    such as arugula, kale, bok choy, collards, or
    spinach, optional, for serving

1. Combine all the ingredients, except the salt, pepper, and greens, in a large pot. Bring to a boil, lower the heat, and simmer for 45 minutes. Season to taste.

NOTE: For even more nutritional benefits, serve over a handful of raw or steamed chopped greens, such as arugula, kale, bok choy, collards, or spinach.

FAST, FILLING CHILI

This almost-instant chili is a great topping for baked potatoes.

▶ SERVES 9

Two 15-ounce cans pinto beans, drained and rinsed

One 15-ounce can diced tomatoes

One 16-ounce jar chunky salsa

⅓ cup textured vegetable protein (see page 232), or 1 veggie
    burger, such as Wildwood or Original Vegan BOCA Burger
    brand, crumbled

2 to 3 teaspoons chili powder, or to taste

1. Combine all the ingredients in large pot and simmer for at least 15 minutes, until the textured vegetable protein is tender.

VARIATIONS: Feel encouraged to add one or more of the following additional ingredients:

- 1 chopped onion
- 1 or more garlic cloves, minced
- 1 seeded, chopped green pepper
- 1 pinch of cumin or cayenne

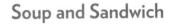

Soup and Sandwich

It's the ultimate comfort combo. Use a ready-made vegan soup or create an impromptu one with whatever you happen to have on hand. Sauté onions and garlic and then add chunks of whatever vegetables strike your fancy. Add vegan vegetable broth and seasonings along with a can of diced tomatoes if you want and leftover beans, pasta, or grains.

Then team your soup up with one of your favorite sandwiches on whole-grain bread (or use one of our suggestions on page 276 or one of the recipes that follow).

SANDWICHES AND SANDWICH SPREADS

MUSHROOM PÂTÉ

Like most sandwich spreads, this one is a multitasker. Serve it on slices of French bread as an hors d'oeuvre, in sandwiches, or on crackers—a perfect side to a soup and salad dinner. It's a also ideal as a make-ahead recipe for parties.

▶ SERVES 6 TO 8

1 tablespoon olive oil
⅔ cup sliced scallions, white and light green parts

1 celery stalk, minced

5 cups diced cremini mushrooms

¾ teaspoon dried herbes de Provence

¼ cup sesame tahini

2 tablespoons low-sodium soy sauce

10 ounces soft silken tofu

1¼ cups fresh whole wheat bread crumbs

½ cup chopped pecans

Dash of cayenne pepper

Freshly ground black pepper, to taste

1. Preheat the oven to 400°F.

2. Heat the oil over medium heat and sauté the scallions and celery until the scallions are tender. Add the mushrooms and herbes de Provence and continue to cook over low heat until the mushrooms are soft.

3. Spoon the mixture into a food processor; add the tahini, soy sauce, tofu, bread crumbs, pecans, cayenne, and black pepper and process them together to the consistency you desire. This doesn't have to be completely smooth. Then taste it and adjust the seasonings.

4. Oil a 9 × 5-inch loaf pan and line it with a piece of wax paper that is several inches larger than the pan. Spoon in the pâté and then fold the wax paper over the top. Bake for 1½ hours.

5. Allow the pâté to cool. Peel back the wax paper and invert the pan to transfer the contents onto a platter. Carefully peel away the wax paper.

RED PEPPER AND WHITE BEAN SPREAD WITH CASHEWS

This spread makes a savory sandwich filling or a festive party dip for raw vegetables. For the sundried tomatoes, use reconstituted, dry tomatoes. Or, if you use tomatoes packed in oil, make sure to drain them first.

▶ MAKES 2½ CUPS

½ large red pepper, seeded and coarsely chopped
1½ cups canned white beans, drained and rinsed
⅓ cup raw cashews
¼ cup chopped sweet onion, such as Texas, Vidalia, or red
1 tablespoon white or yellow miso
1 tablespoon Dijon mustard
¼ cup sun-dried tomatoes

1. Combine all the ingredients in a food processor and process until smooth.

5 SANDWICHES FOR THE SANDWICH GENERATION

1. **Create a veggie sub.** Use any combination of lettuce or other greens, tomato, avocado, hummus, red pepper, fennel, green pepper, mushrooms, red cabbage, cucumber, olives, sprouts, celery, carrots, radishes, radicchio, arugula, mashed beans, onions, sprouts, baked tofu, and vegan versions of turkey, chicken, bologna, bacon, or sausage. Buy or make some vegan meatballs and you can even have a veggie meatball sandwich.

2. **Order a veggie sandwich at a sandwich place, such as Subway.** Hold the mayo!

3. **Try a grilled cheese sandwich made with Daiya brand or another meltable vegan cheese**, or use Dragonfly's Bulk Dry Uncheese Mix (page 224).

4. **Don't forget peanut butter:** A sandwich of peanut or almond butter with a sliced banana, lettuce, or jelly is a childhood favorite that is still a taste treat decades after we may have enjoyed one. (For a change, grill the sandwich.)

5. **Veganize your favorite sandwiches.** Patti makes a BLT using Smart Bacon, a vegan bacon substitute.

BBQ "BEEF" SANDWICHES WITH BEEF-STYLE SEITAN

Seitan can satisfy anybody's craving for meat. You can buy it prepared or make your own using this easy recipe that was shared with us by Eddie Garza of Mercy for Animals. (We also provide a more complex seitan recipe perfected by Sandy Weiland on page 231.) If you are using homemade BBQ sauce and seitan, each needs to be refrigerated overnight, so begin the day before you will be serving the sandwiches. If you are going the quick route with store-bought BBQ sauce and seitan, you can jump directly to step 5, which calls for sautéing the seitan and adding the BBQ sauce.

▶ MAKES 6 SANDWICHES

Seitan:

4 cubes vegan beef-style bouillon (see box on page 285)

1 tablespoon sesame tahini

1 teaspoon vegan Worcestershire sauce

1 teaspoon liquid smoke

1 cup vital wheat gluten

2 teaspoons vegetable oil

BBQ Sauce:

¼ cup coarsely chopped onion

3 garlic cloves, peeled

One 15-ounce can tomato sauce

1 tablespoon canola oil

2 tablespoons liquid smoke

¼ cup cider vinegar

¼ cup molasses

¼ cup evaporated cane sweetener

1 tablespoon vegan Worcestershire sauce

2 teaspoons hot pepper sauce, such as Tabasco

1 teaspoon freshly ground black pepper

¼ teaspoon cayenne pepper, optional (not really!)

Sandwiches:

> 12 slices of bread
>
> Vegan mayo
>
> Pickles

1. To prepare the seitan, combine one of the bouillon cubes with the tahini, Worcestershire sauce, liquid smoke, and ¾ cup of warm water in a large bowl. Mix well. Add the wheat gluten and knead the mixture until well combined.

2. Cut the prepared wheat gluten (now properly referred to as seitan) into six equal chunks.

3. Bring 6 cups of water to a boil and add the remaining 3 bouillon cubes. Place the seitan into the boiling broth, lower the heat, and simmer for 45 minutes. Drain and refrigerate overnight.

4. Prepare the sauce: Purée the onion, garlic, and tomato sauce in a food processor. Combine the puree, all the remaining sauce ingredients, and ¼ cup of water in a large saucepan. Simmer over low heat for 30 to 45 minutes, whisking often. Refrigerate the sauce overnight.

5. Cut the seitan chunks into thin slices. Heat the vegetable oil in a large skillet over medium-high heat and sauté the slices until almost crisp. Pour the entire batch of BBQ sauce over the seitan, and lower the heat. Simmer the seitan in the sauce on low heat for 10 to 15 minutes, stirring occasionally.

6. To assemble the sandwiches, lightly grill or toast the bread. Dress 6 of the slices with vegan mayo and pickles, and the other six with the BBQ sauce–seitan mixture.

BEEF-STYLE BOUILLON

MANY BOUILLON PRODUCTS OFFER a beef-like flavor. A popular vegan brand is Better than Bouillon, which has a vegan vegetable base and is thick and creamy. It can be added to soups in place of beef stock. A chicken-flavored vegan vegetable bouillon is also available from the same company. Better than Bouillon is stocked in supermarkets with other broth and stocks.

Edward & Sons makes a beef-style vegan bouillon cube that could be used in the above "beef" sandwiches. If you cannot find the cubes, substitute a teaspoon of Better than Bouillon for each cube the recipe calls for.

PHILLY CHEESESTEAK

YOU CAN USE SEITAN to make Philly cheesesteaks. Simply marinate seitan in some vegan Worcestershire sauce, and add caramelized onions and peppers, vegan mozzarella, and a spicy mayo! (To caramelize onions, fry them slowly for a long time, until they are slightly browned.)

GROOVIN' REUBEN

This is one of those recipes that was passed around so many times, Carol says she can't recall who gave it to her first. But it carried the title "Groovin' Reuben"—which we think is a great description. Carol's twenty-something son, Ben, makes huge amounts of it. (The title also inspired him to write a poem in its honor.) Carol and Ben prepared it for a meat-eating college friend of Ben's, who declared that it was the best Reuben he'd had. Because these are so popular, and the leftovers are just as good, we always double the recipe. If you decide to do the same, you will need to use two pans to hold the number of tempeh pieces.

▶ MAKES 4 SANDWICHES

8 ounces tempeh, sliced in half horizontally, and then each slice divided into 4 parts
3 tablespoons extra virgin olive oil
3 tablespoons tamari
1 cup sauerkraut
8 vegan cheese slices
8 slices toasted rye bread

Dressing:

    3 tablespoons vegan mayonnaise

    2 tablespoons ketchup

    2 tablespoons dill pickle relish

    1 teaspoon cider vinegar

    ¼ teaspoon sea salt

    Pinch of freshly ground black pepper

1. Steam the tempeh for 20 minutes. In a shallow dish, combine the olive oil, tamari, and 2 tablespoons of water. Add the steamed tempeh and marinate for about an hour. Remove the tempeh from the marinade. Pour the marinade into an iron or stainless-steel skillet and heat until warm.

2. When the marinade is warm, add the tempeh, cover, and cook over medium-low heat for 5 to 8 minutes, turning once. Arrange the sauerkraut over the tempeh, followed by the vegan cheese slices. You may need to add a couple of tablespoons of water to the skillet if the marinade has been absorbed. Cover and cook over low heat for 2 to 3 minutes more, or until the cheese melts.

3. To make the dressing, whisk all the dressing ingredients together.

4. Lightly toast the bread and add some dressing to each side. Then add the tempeh mixture, and enjoy!

VEGETABLE DISHES

ROASTED VEGGIES AND TOFU

Roasting veggies is an easy and delicious way to prepare them. Because you can serve them hot out of the oven or at room temperature, they provide flexibility in serving. Feel free to use whichever vegetables you have on hand or that have the most appeal to you. You can line any baking sheet with parchment paper to create a nonstick surface, making cleanup easier. Serve them in a colorful pie plate or pottery bowl if you have one.

A successful and colorful meal could be made using a variety of roasted veggies, baked tofu, and a large salad.

▶ **SERVES 6**

Vegetable possibilities:
> Carrots, cut into ¼-inch slices
> Brussels sprouts, sliced in half if their diameter is larger than a quarter
> Cauliflower, broken into florets
> Broccoli, trimmed, stalks peeled and sliced, florets separated
> Butternut squash, peeled, seeded, and cubed (grocery stores often sell pre-cubed winter squash)
> Red onions
> Sliced eggplant
> Tomatoes
> Extra-firm tofu
> Bok choy (10 minutes' roasting time)
> Asparagus (10 minutes' roasting time)
> Portobello mushrooms, left whole (10 minutes' roasting time)

Basic preparation:
> 2 pounds vegetables or tofu, cubed
> 2 tablespoons olive oil
> 1 teaspoon salt
> ½ teaspoon freshly ground black pepper

1. Preheat the oven to 400°F.

2. In a large, bowl, toss the prepared veggies or tofu with the oil, salt, and pepper. Arrange on a baking sheet.

3. Roast the bok choy, asparagus, and portobello mushrooms only for 10 minutes. Prick with a fork to check for tenderness, then remove from the oven.

4. For all other veggies and tofu, bake for 15 minutes. Shake the pan to dislodge the veggies and turn them over so that they brown evenly. Return to the oven to roast for another 15 minutes, or until crunchy outside and soft inside.

SUGGESTED PREPARATIONS

- Brussels sprouts: After removing from the oven, toss with poppy seeds and 1 tablespoon tamari.
- Tofu: After 15 minutes of roasting, toss with ½ teaspoon garlic powder, ½ teaspoon ground ginger, and 2 tablespoons nutritional yeast. Flip over and roast for another 10 minutes. Toss with 1 tablespoon tamari.
- Cauliflower: Roasted with 15 whole garlic cloves.
- A mixture of butternut squash, carrots, and red onion: After removing from the oven, toss with 2 tablespoons fennel seeds and 1 tablespoon balsamic vinegar.
- Bok choy: After removing from the oven, toss with vegetarian oyster sauce (available in Chinese grocery stores).

SPICY COLLARDS WITH GINGER

Even if collard greens have never been a part of your family dinners, now's the time to consider trying them. This Southern staple is rich in calcium and vitamin A and also contains a host of disease-fighting phytochemicals. In this recipe, we've flavored the collards with a bit of hot pepper—a traditional way to season them in some parts of Africa where they are a commonly consumed vegetable—and some grated fresh ginger.

▶ SERVES 4

2 cups vegan vegetable stock or broth
1 pound collards
1 tablespoon extra virgin olive oil
¾ cup coarsely chopped onion
1 garlic clove, minced

1 tablespoon grated fresh ginger, or 1 teaspoon ground
¼ teaspoon cayenne, or to taste
Salt and freshly ground black pepper

1. Bring the vegetable stock to a boil in a large sauce pan. Tear the collard leaves into small pieces, discarding the stems. Add to the stock and simmer for 15 minutes, until tender.

2. Heat the olive oil in a skillet over medium heat. Add the onion and garlic and sauté until the onion is just tender. Add the ginger and cayenne and stir for 1 minute.

3. Drain the collards and add to the onion. Stir over low heat until the collards are mixed well with the onion, garlic, and seasonings. Season with salt and pepper.

KALE WITH CINNAMON

The spicy sweetness of cinnamon tempers the slightly bitter flavor of kale. It's a great way to get to know this nutrient-packed vegetable.

▶ **SERVES 4 TO 6**

1 tablespoon canola or soybean oil
½ cup minced onion
1 garlic clove , minced
⅛ teaspoon ground cinnamon
1 pound raw kale, washed, stems removed, and coarsely chopped
1 teaspoon red wine vinegar
Salt and freshly ground black pepper

1. Heat the oil in a large, deep stockpot over medium heat. Add the onion and sauté for 5 minutes. Add the garlic and cinnamon and sauté for another 2 minutes. Add the kale and toss to coat with the cinnamon mixture. Add 1 cup of water, cover, and simmer over low heat for 15 minutes.

2. Remove from the heat and drain off any excess cooking water. Add the vinegar and toss to combine. Season with salt and pepper.

GREENS AND MUSHROOMS

This simple dish is fine by itself and terrific served over baked potatoes, rice, or quinoa. Many markets sell prewashed, presliced mushrooms that will make this dish even quicker to prepare.

▶ **SERVES 2**

> 1 bunch kale, collards, or chard, stems removed
>   7 to 10 large leaves)
> ¼ cup vegan vegetable stock or broth or water, or more as
>   needed
> 1 red or yellow onion, halved and sliced
> 1 cup cleaned and sliced mushrooms
> 1 teaspoon soy sauce, or to taste

1. Wash the greens and chop them into bite-size pieces. (There is no need to dry them.)
2. Heat the stock in a skillet or pot. Add the onion and sauté until it just starts to turn transparent, about 3 minutes. (If needed, add more water, a little at a time.)
3. Add the mushrooms and cook for another 3 minutes, stirring frequently. Add the greens and continue to cook for another 3 minutes, stirring frequently. Add the soy sauce, mix together, and serve.

SWEET AND SOUR RED CABBAGE

This is another of Shirley Wilkes-Johnson's wonderful recipes. Serve with just a dollop of vegan sour cream on top.

▶ **SERVES 6**

2 tablespoons vegan margarine

1 head red cabbage, halved, cored, and chopped coarsely

1 cup chopped onion

1 apple, peeled, cored, and chopped

¼ cup sugar

⅓ cup balsamic vinegar

1 tablespoon tamari

½ teaspoon salt, or to taste

¼ teaspoon freshly ground black pepper

1. Melt the margarine in a pot that's large enough to hold the cabbage. Add the cabbage, onion, and apple and sauté together over medium-high heat for about 5 minutes. Add the sugar and toss the mixture to coat. Stir in the vinegar, tamari, salt, and pepper. Cover and simmer for 30 to 35 minutes. Pierce the cabbage with a fork to determine its softness.

MASHED POTATOES AND GRAVY

This is one of the most popular recipes created by Jennifer Raymond—American traditional fare, made vegan, at its finest! Serve with Neatloaf (page 310) for a meal that will satisfy even the most committed carnivore!

▶ **SERVES 6 TO 8**

4 large russet potatoes, peeled and diced

½ teaspoon salt, plus more as needed

½ to 1 cup soy or rice milk

½ teaspoon toasted sesame oil, or 1 teaspoon olive oil

1 small onion, chopped (about ½ cup)

1 cup thinly sliced cremini mushrooms

1 tablespoon unbleached all-purpose flour

1 tablespoon soy sauce

¼ teaspoon freshly ground black pepper

1. Place the potatoes in a pot with 2 cups of water and the ½ teaspoon of salt. Bring to a boil, lower the heat, and simmer until tender, 15 to 20 minutes. Drain and reserve the liquid. Mash the potatoes, then add enough soy or rice milk to make the potatoes creamy. Add salt to taste. Transfer to a serving bowl, cover, and set aside.

2. Heat the oil in a large skillet and sauté the onion and mushrooms over high heat, stirring frequently, until browned, about 5 minutes.

3. Return the potato cooking water to the pot and whisk in the flour, soy sauce, and pepper. Add the onion mixture and cook over medium heat, stirring constantly, until thick. If you prefer smooth gravy, puree it in a blender. Be sure to start on low speed and hold the lid on tightly.

4. Transfer the gravy to a gravy bowl and serve with the mashed potatoes.

WHITE BEAN GRAVY WITH GINGER AND CINNAMON

If you are looking for a nutritious variation on the traditional gravy found in the previous recipe, try this one. Cooked white beans add fiber and protein to this ginger- and cinnamon-flavored gravy from JL Fields, who blogs at JLGoesVegan.com and is the coauthor with Ginny of *Vegan for Her*. Serve the gravy over rice or old-fashioned mashed potatoes (see the previous recipe for mashed potatoes).

▶ **MAKES 3 TO 4 CUPS**

4 tablespoons (½ stick) vegan margarine
½ cup chopped yellow onion
⅛ teaspoon ground ginger
⅛ teaspoon ground cinnamon
⅛ teaspoon freshly ground black pepper
1¼ cups vegan vegetable stock or broth
¼ cup low-sodium soy sauce

1½ cups cooked small white beans, or one 15-ounce can, drained
   and rinsed

2 tablespoons nutritional yeast

1. Melt the margarine in a saucepan over medium-high heat. Add the onion and sauté until translucent.

2. Add the ginger, cinnamon, and pepper and stir well. Stir in the veggie stock and soy sauce and return to a boil. Add the beans.

3. Use an immersion blender to blend the gravy, 20 to 30 seconds. (You can also use a regular blender; simply return the gravy back to the saucepan once it's blended.)

4. Cover, lower the heat to medium, and cook for 5 minutes, stirring occasionally. Add the nutritional yeast, stir well, cover, and simmer for 5 more minutes, stirring as needed.

YUM PUK GOOD (THAI-STYLE ASPARAGUS)

This dish is traditionally made with wild ferns, but outside Thailand asparagus is much more available. To trim asparagus, bend it from the bottom till it breaks apart. Alternatively, simply cut away the ends.

▶ SERVES 4

10 ounces trimmed asparagus

2 tablespoons roasted peanuts, coarsely ground

2 ounces extra-firm tofu, pureed

¼ cup fresh lime juice

1 teaspoon salt

1 teaspoon sugar

3 tablespoons coconut milk

1. Have ready a bowl of cold water.

2. Cook the asparagus in a small skillet of boiling water for 2 minutes. Transfer to the bowl of cold water.

3. Mix together all the remaining ingredients in a separate bowl. Drain the asparagus, add to the sauce, and toss to combine.

TSIMMIS (HOLIDAY BAKED YAM CASSEROLE)

Because *tsimmis* has so many ingredients, the expression "Don't make a *tsimmis*" has come to mean to not make a big deal out of something. This traditional, sweet casserole is a staple at Passover and other holiday meals. It takes 90 minutes to bake, but once it's in the oven, your job is nearly over! To save time, look for peeled and chopped squash, which is available in many markets.

▶ **SERVES 8 AS A SIDE DISH**

1 small butternut squash
3 large yams, peeled, and cut into chunks
1 apple, cored and diced
4 large carrots, peeled and cut into chunks
¼ cup dark raisins
¼ cup light raisins
¼ cup dates, pitted and diced
Three 2- to 3-inch cinnamon sticks
2 tablespoons organic sugar (see box on page 228)
Finely grated zest and juice of 1 orange
Rind of 1 orange, chopped about ¼ inch thick and 2 inches long
¼ cup pure maple syrup

1. Preheat the oven to 350°F.
2. Prepare the squash by peeling, seeding, and dicing it. (For an easier way to prepare the squash, bake the whole squash—check it at 30 minutes by pricking it with a fork to make sure it is tender—and then let it cool before peeling, halving, and seeding it.)
3. Place the yams, apples, carrots, and squash in a baking dish. Add the two kinds of raisins and the dates, cinnamon sticks, and sugar.

Add the orange zest, juice, and rind, and maple syrup and combine well.

4. Bake for 30 minutes. Stir, then bake for another 30 minutes. Stir one more time and bake for another 30 minutes. (The total baking time is 90 minutes.) Remove from the oven, remove the cinnamon sticks, and serve.

SPICE MIXES, BEANS, AND GRAINS

Beans and grains sit at the center of many vegan plates, and vegans never get tired of them because there are so many different types.

DRIED AND CANNED BEANS

You'll find black, navy, garbanzo, kidney, pinto, white beans, and lima beans, plus lentils, black-eyed peas, and split peas in most grocery stores. For fast meals or picnics, look for vegetarian baked beans. Check specialty stores for some other interesting options like little red adzuki beans, maroon and white speckled Anasazi beans, and mung beans.

GRAINS

You already know about oats and brown rice, but there are many other whole grains that can give your meals added interest and international flair. Each has its own unique taste and texture. Because grains have a long shelf life, you can keep lots of different ones on hand. Here are a few that you can find in most grocery stores:

Barley: One of the oldest domesticated foods in the world, barley has a chewy quality and mild taste. It is very high in soluble fiber and is a good choice if you need to lower your cholesterol. Pearled barley has the outer bran removed and cooks more quickly but is still high in fiber.

Bulgur: A fast-food type of grain, this is whole wheat that has been precooked and then dried. It's common in Middle Eastern cooking where it's used to make the classic dish tabbouleh.

Couscous: Common in the cuisines of North Africa, this is made from steamed, dried wheat and it cooks very quickly. Although the traditional couscous is a refined grain, you can find whole wheat couscous.

Quinoa: This high-protein grain was a staple in the diet of the Incans, who called it the "mother grain." Quinoa is fast cooking, which has made it very popular among modern cooks.

Wheat berries: A slow-cooking grain with a very chewy quality; wheat berries are usually mixed with other grains.

COOKING TIMES FOR GRAINS

For each cup of dry grain, use 2 cups of water.*

*Barley, hulled	1½ hours
Barley, pearled	50 minutes
Couscous	5 minutes
Kamut	45 minutes
Quinoa	15 minutes
Rice, white	20 minutes
Rice, brown	40 minutes
Spelt	45 minutes
*Wheat berries	2 hours

*Because hulled barley and wheat berries take a long time to cook, some of the water will evaporate in the process. Therefore you may wish to start with 3 cups water to 1 cup of grain.

SPICE OPTIONS FOR GRAINS AND LEGUMES

These spice mixtures first appeared in *VegEasy*, a collection of over 225 animal-free recipes published in 2003 by the Dallas-based Vegetarian Education Network (VegNet). As with many of the other recipes found in this book, these mixtures provide a way to try different flavors. You can cook big pots of lentils and brown rice and season portions with a different spice mix each night of the week. Not only do these mixtures provide you with choices in flavors, they can be made in minutes. Now you'll be able to prepare easy meals that have an international flair whenever you want.

CHINESE FIVE-SPICE SEASONING

1 tablespoon ground star anise
1 tablespoon ground Szechuan pepper
1½ teaspoons ground cassia or cinnamon
1 tablespoon ground fennel seeds
1½ teaspoons ground cloves

1. Combine the spices in a jar and shake well to combine. Store in an airtight jar.

CREOLE SEASONING

1 teaspoon cayenne pepper
2 tablespoons freshly ground white pepper
2 tablespoons freshly ground black pepper
1 tablespoon salt
1 tablespoon garlic powder
½ teaspoon ground celery seeds
2 teaspoons dried oregano
1½ teaspoons dried thyme

1. Combine the spices in a jar and shake well to combine. Store in an airtight jar.

HERBES DE PROVENCE

1 tablespoon dried basil

1½ teaspoons dried marjoram

1 tablespoon dried chervil

1 teaspoon dried tarragon

2 tablespoons dried thyme

1 tablespoon dried summer savory

1 teaspoon dried culinary-grade lavender

1 tablespoon dried rosemary

1 teaspoon dried mint

½ teaspoon dried oregano

1. Combine the herbs in a jar and shake well to combine. Store in an airtight jar. You can grind the seasoning mix in a clean coffee grinder, if you prefer it to be finer.

GREEK SEASONINGS

2 tablespoons dried oregano

¼ cup dried parsley

1 tablespoon dried thyme

2 teaspoons garlic powder

1. Combine the herbs in a jar and shake well to combine. Store in an airtight jar.

MILD INDIAN CURRY SEASONING

This recipe produces a very mild curry mixture. If you wish to turn up the fire, add more pepper, of course. You might also add more ginger.

1 teaspoon garlic powder

1 teaspoon ground ginger

1 teaspoon ground turmeric

½ teaspoon ground allspice

½ teaspoon ground coriander

½ teaspoon ground fenugreek

½ teaspoon dry mustard

¼ teaspoon freshly ground black pepper

¼ teaspoon ground red pepper

1. Combine the spices in a jar and shake well to combine. Store in an airtight jar.

ITALIAN SEASONING

Although Italian cuisine rarely incorporates dried herbs, this mix is dried, for convenience. "Italian seasoning" is so popular as a mixture, it is sold commercially; but you can make it yourself.

2 teaspoons dried parsley

2 teaspoons dried oregano

1 tablespoon dried basil

2 teaspoons dried rosemary

1 teaspoon dried marjoram

½ teaspoon dried sage

1. Combine the herbs in a jar and shake well to combine. Store in an airtight jar.

JAMAICAN HEAT WAVE SPICE

1 teaspoon garlic powder

1 teaspoon ground ginger

1 teaspoon mustard seeds

1 teaspoon onion powder

½ teaspoon ground allspice

½ teaspoon ground cloves

½ teaspoon paprika

½ teaspoon dried thyme

½ teaspoon red pepper flakes

½ teaspoon black peppercorns

1. Combine the spices in a small bowl, then grind in a coffee grinder. Store in an airtight jar.

COOKING DRIED BEANS

Some beans (lentils and split peas) never need presoaking. Others, such as soybeans, favas, and chickpeas, will cook better if you soak them first. For all other beans, such as kidney beans, black beans, navy beans, and pinto beans, soaking is optional. See page 89 for the pros and cons of presoaking beans. In short, if beans give you gas, then soaking will help alleviate that problem. If not, then you don't need to bother.

To soak beans, rinse them first, then place in a large bowl with 3 cups of water for every cup of dried beans (or 6 cups of water per pound). Refrigerate for at least 4 hours. Drain and rinse the beans.

To cook, place the beans in a large pot and add 3 cups of water or broth for each cup of dried beans you started out with. Bring the water to a boil, lower the heat to simmer, and cook the beans until they're tender—1 to 2 hours, depending on the type of bean.

You can also cook beans in your slow cooker. Place the soaked or unsoaked beans in the cooker along with enough water or vegan stock to cover the beans, plus an inch or two more. Cook on low overnight or on high for 3 to 4 hours, until beans are tender. Add chopped onions and any seasoning you like at the beginning of the cooking time to produce a kitchen filled with wonderful aromas and a meal that is ready when you need it.

COOKING TIMES FOR DRIED BEANS

BEAN	COOKING TIME FOR SOAKED BEANS	COOKING TIME FOR UNSOAKED BEANS
Adzuki	1½ hours	2 to 3 hours
Black	1½ to 2 hours	2 to 3 hours
Black-eyed peas	½ hour	1 hour
Cannellini	1 to 1½ hours	2 hours
Chickpeas	2 hours	3½ to 4 hours
Great northern	1½ to 2 hours	2 to 3 hours
Kidney	1½ to 2 hours	2 to 3 hours
Lentils		½ to ¾ hour
Lima, baby	¾ to 1 hour	1½ hours
Navy	1½ to 2 hours	2 to 3 hours
Pinto	1½ to 2 hours	2 to 3 hours
Soybeans	2 to 3 hours	3 to 4 hours
Split peas		¾ hour

HEAT WAVE BEANS

Turn up the heat on this simple rice and bean dish and taste the difference the spice mixture makes.

▶ SERVES 4

2 cups cooked red kidney beans, or one 15-ounce can, drained and rinsed

1 cup coconut milk

2 cups uncooked brown rice

1 teaspoon salt

1 tablespoon Jamaican Heat Wave Spice (page 294), or to taste

Lemon wedges, for serving

1. Combine all the ingredients plus 3 cups of water in a saucepan, cover, and bring to a simmer over medium-high heat. Lower the heat and simmer until the liquid is absorbed and grains of rice have separated, about 40 minutes. Stir before serving to distribute the beans evenly. Serve with lemon wedges and offer additional Jamaican Heat Wave Spice at your table for those who really want to turn up the heat.

ALMOND-MISO SAUCE

Because the composition of miso automatically adds the savory flavor of umami (see page 49) to this sauce, JL Fields, coauthor with Ginny of *Vegan for Her,* says it's a great choice to bridge the "vegan-omnivore gap" when cooking for a mixed crowd. She serves it over "hippie bowls" of grains, beans, and greens.

MAKES ABOUT ⅔ CUP

⅔ cup raw unsalted almonds

2 tablespoons yellow miso

¼ teaspoon garlic powder

1. Combine all the ingredients plus ¼ cup of water in a blender. Blend for 2 to 3 minutes and add more water, if necessary, to achieve a thick sauce.

FESTIVE QUINOA

This beautiful quinoa dish is perfect for holiday celebrations. The pale yellow grain is a lovely backdrop for the red, green, and black ingredients.

▶ **SERVES 4 TO 6**

1 cup quinoa, rinsed (see note on page 264)
3 cups kale (any kind), cut or torn into bite-size pieces
½ cup sun-dried tomatoes, chopped (see note)
¾ cup black olives, pitted and halved or sliced

1. Bring 2 cups of water to a boil in a medium saucepan. Add the quinoa and lower the heat to a simmer. Cook for 10 minutes. Add the kale and cook for an additional 2 minutes, or until the water is absorbed by the quinoa.
2. Transfer the quinoa to a bowl and add the tomatoes and olives. Toss and serve.

NOTE: Sun-dried tomatoes come marinated in oil in a jar, or dried in bulk or in packages. If you are buying the tomatoes dried, place them in a bowl and pour boiling water over them. Let them sit in the water for 15 minutes to soften. Drain and chop each dried piece into two or three pieces.

CHRISTINA'S BLACK-BEAN BURGERS WITH MANGO BBQ SAUCE

Carol's friend Christina (see page 226 for more on Christina's vegan cooking) made ninety of these sliders (or mini burgers) for her niece's wedding rehearsal dinner picnic. They are spicy and tender, and their Southwestern flavor makes them irresistible. The mango sauce (adapted from Lukas Volger's book *Veggie Burgers Every Which Way*) adds a kick! The burger mixture can separate if you're not careful, so freeze them for at least 30 minutes before cooking. The freezing firms them up so they won't fall apart (at least as much) when you cook them.

▶ **MAKES 6 TO 8 REGULAR-SIZE BURGERS OR 12 TO 15 SLIDERS**

Mango BBQ Sauce (makes 2 cups):
  1 cup ketchup
  ¾ cup mango chutney
  ½ cup cider vinegar
  2 teaspoons Dijon mustard
  1 teaspoon chili powder
  1 teaspoon liquid smoke
  1 tablespoon molasses
  2 garlic cloves, minced
  1 tablespoon grated onion
  ¼ teaspoon cayenne pepper

Burgers:
  4 tablespoons extra virgin olive oil
  1 yellow onion, diced small
  One 14-ounce can black beans, drained and rinsed
  1 small carrot, finely shredded (about ½ cup)
  ⅓ cup cornmeal
  ⅓ cup bread crumbs
  1 tablespoon chili powder
  1 teaspoon sea salt
  ½ cup finely chopped fresh cilantro
  6 to 8 regular buns or 12 to 15 slider buns
  Shredded lettuce and sliced tomatoes

1. Prepare the sauce: Bring ⅓ cup of water and all of the sauce ingredients to a boil in a medium saucepan. Lower the heat and simmer over very low heat for 15 minutes. Refrigerate any leftover sauce for up to 2 weeks.

2. Prepare the burgers: Heat 2 tablespoons of the olive oil in a large skillet over medium heat. Add the onion and sauté until tender and slightly caramelized, about 20 minutes.

3. Mash together the onions, beans, carrot, cornmeal, bread crumbs, chili powder, salt, cilantro, and ⅓ cup of water in a large bowl. Use a large spoon, or even your hands, to do the job. Use your hands to form the mixture into 6 to 8 regular-size patties or 12 to 15 slider-size patties. Refrigerate for 20 minutes (or freeze for later use).

4. Heat the remaining 2 tablespoons olive oil in a large nonstick skillet over medium high heat. Add the patties and let each brown on one side before flipping (about 3 minutes for each side), adding more olive oil to the skillet as needed.

5. Toast the buns, add the patties and garnish the burgers with shredded lettuce, a slice of tomato, and a generous portion of Mango BBQ Sauce.

BEANS AND GREENS

This recipe is from Colleen Welsh (see interview, page 15), who writes, "To make this a meal, I add Field Roast or Tofurky Italian sausage that has been sliced and browned. Add it after the beans . . . yum!"

▶ **SERVES 4**

2 tablespoons extra virgin olive oil

3 garlic cloves, minced

2 bunches greens (such as kale, escarole, or Swiss chard), stems removed, torn into bite-size pieces

One 15-ounce can cannellini or any white bean of your choice, drained and rinsed

Pinch red pepper flakes, optional

Salt and freshly ground black pepper

1. Heat the olive oil in a large skillet over medium-high heat. Add the garlic and sauté, until browned. Add the greens gradually and sauté until wilted. Add the beans and red pepper flakes. (If you don't like hot food, omit the pepper flakes.) Heat through and add salt and black pepper to taste. Serve with crusty, rustic bread.

MAIN-COURSE MEALS

You may prefer to have heavier meals in the morning and lighter ones later in the day. Or perhaps you prefer all light meals—grazing throughout the day.

No matter when you eat the meal you think of as "dinner," the following pages contain a variety of choices for you to try for your main meal of the day. According to some reports, the average family actually eats only ten different dinner meals. Of those ten basic meals, some probably are flexible enough to be veganized easily. Spaghetti and meat balls could become spaghetti in a mushroom sauce, spaghetti with veggie meatballs, spaghetti with textured vegetable protein. Keep your favorite lasagna recipes (or use our recipe, page 303). Either way, use our ricotta cheese (page 223) or Parmesan (page 224).

Stuffed peppers? Replace the meat with chopped portobello mushrooms, or veggie ground beef, the dairy cheese with nondairy Cheddar cheese, and add the usual tomatoes and onions.

Pizzas? At a pizza place that doesn't have vegan cheese, a slight dash of red wine vinegar on top of the pizza will give it a sharpness that others might be getting by spooning Parmesan cheese on top of their pizza. Top the pizza with mushrooms, garlic, onions, olives, and any other veggies that are offered.

"CHICKEN" PICCATA

This is another recipe from Colleen Welsh, who says she likes to serve the "chicken" with pasta or rice and spoon the sauce over the cutlets. Garnish with a lemon slice and fresh parsley and pair with roasted or grilled asparagus.

▶ SERVES 4

One 10-ounce package Gardein Chick'n Scallopini—defrosted
    and molded slightly to look like 4 chicken cutlets
Nondairy milk, as needed
Whole wheat flour, as needed
2 tablespoons olive oil or, if preferred, vegan margarine
2 garlic cloves, minced
½ cup white wine
Juice of 1 lemon
3 tablespoons capers

1. Dip the cutlets in the nondairy milk and then dredge them in the flour. Heat the olive oil in a large skillet. Add the cutlets and cook in a skillet until both sides are well browned, 3 to 5 minutes per side. Assemble them on a platter. Add the garlic to the skillet and cook it until lightly browned. Deglaze the pan with white wine and add the lemon juice and capers. Reduce until the sauce is slightly thickened. Return the cutlets to the pan and cook for 2 minutes.

NOTE: Gardein Chick'n is a relatively new product that has become extremely popular, so much so that many supermarkets can be found carrying it in their frozen food section. Look for the "natural" or "organic" or "meat substitute" section of the frozen food department, or ask for it to be stocked. Besides trying Colleen's "Chicken" Piccata recipe, you can bake this Chick'n and make chick'n sandwiches with it.

HELEN R. MOY'S MAC AND CHEESE

It's hard to find anyone who doesn't love mac and cheese. After Donald Moy (page 180) raved about his mom's mac and cheese, we wanted to provide the recipe so others could enjoy it as well. The ground cashews provide a creaminess and the nutritional yeast provides the Cheddar-y taste.

▶ **SERVES 6 TO 8**

1 cup unsweetened soy milk

2 cups raw, unsalted cashews

14 ounces whole wheat macaroni

½ cup diced seeded red bell pepper (fresh or roasted)

¼ cup nutritional yeast

2 tablespoons fresh lemon juice

1 teaspoon salt

2 teaspoons onion powder

2 teaspoons garlic powder

1 tablespoon paprika

¼ cup vegetable oil

1 teaspoon sugar

1. Combine the soy milk and cashews in a blender and let soak for at least an hour to soften the cashews.

2. Preheat the oven to 375°F. Oil a baking dish. Boil the macaroni according to the package directions, until tender. Drain the cooked macaroni.

3. Blend the cashews. Add all the remaining ingredients to the blender and blend until the contents become a smooth sauce.

4. Mix together the sauce and the macaroni and pour into the prepared baking dish. Bake for 20 to 30 minutes, until the top is browned.

LASAGNA

Many lasagna recipes take a long time to prepare. This one saves time by using tomato sauce from a jar and by not precooking the noodles. The extra water helps the noodles cook while they are baking. If you want to "doctor" the jar of sauce, add anything you like: mushrooms, garlic, more oregano, basil, onion, sun-dried tomatoes. If you make the tofu ricotta in advance, you'll save an additional 5 minutes.

One of the benefits of vegan cooking: most recipes are very forgiving. While it's difficult to make lasagna without tomato sauce, noodles, and some sort of cheese layer, virtually every other ingredient is optional. So if you don't have zucchini, you can still make the recipe. You can substitute diced peppers or mushrooms or grated carrots, or just skip that ingredient altogether. Carol uses sliced, sautéed portobello mushrooms. The same goes for the garlic, oregano, spinach, and paprika. And if you don't have tofu, but you happen to have a commercial vegan cheese in the fridge, use what you have. Don't skip a recipe just because you're missing one or two ingredients. By improvising and experimenting you make the recipe your own! This recipe first appeared in Carol and Patti's book, *How to Eat Like a Vegetarian Even if You Never Want to Be One.*

▶ **MAKES ONE 9 X 13-INCH PAN; SERVES 8 TO 10**

One 24- or 25-ounce jar vegan tomato sauce
1 package lasagna noodles (whole wheat, if available)
1 batch Tofu Ricotta (page 223)
1 zucchini, grated
One 16-ounce package frozen chopped spinach, thawed
1 tablespoon dried oregano
2 or more garlic cloves, minced, optional
2 teaspoons paprika

1. Preheat the oven to 350°F.
2. Mix 1½ cups of water and the tomato sauce to make a thinner sauce.

3. Ladle a layer of the thin tomato sauce on the bottom of a 9 × 13-inch baking dish.

4. Cover with a layer of noodles. (Usually, you will have to break some noodles so they fit all the way to the edges of the pan.)

5. Sprinkle the tofu ricotta evenly over the noodles. (Don't try to be too even-handed; it will be unevenly covered, and that's okay.)

6. Sprinkle half of the grated zucchini and half of the thawed spinach over the ricotta layer.

7. Sprinkle half of the oregano and half of the garlic (if using) over this layer.

8. Add a generous layer of the tomato sauce, and another layer of noodles.

9. Repeat the layers of tofu ricotta, zucchini, spinach, oregano, garlic, and tomato sauce, ending with noodles on top covered with tomato sauce and a little tofu ricotta.

10. Sprinkle the paprika over the whole dish.

11. Cover with parchment paper and foil, and bake for 35 minutes. Uncover and bake for an additional 10 to 15 minutes.

TEMPEH AND VEGETABLES WITH INDONESIAN PEANUT SAUCE

Protein-rich tempeh, a fermented soy food, is a staple of Indonesian cuisine. We've paired it with Indonesian peanut sauce and lots of colorful vegetables. For this recipe, you can substitute whatever vegetables you like.

▶ SERVES 4

Indonesian Peanut Sauce:
1 tablespoon brown sugar
1 tablespoon fresh lemon juice
¼ cup natural peanut butter
1 teaspoon hot pepper sauce, or to taste

Tempeh and Vegetables:

>2 tablespoons canola or peanut oil
>
>8 ounces tempeh, cut into ½-inch cubes
>
>4 garlic cloves, minced
>
>2 cups thinly sliced carrots
>
>1 red bell pepper, seeded and cut into strips
>
>½ pound broccoli, chopped into small florets
>
>½ cup sliced scallions, white and light green parts

1. To prepare the sauce, place ¼ cup of water in a small saucepan and add the brown sugar, lemon juice, peanut butter, and hot pepper sauce. Stir with a whisk to combine over low heat until smooth and hot. Let cook over very low heat while you prepare the tempeh and vegetables.

2. To prepare the tempeh and vegetables: Heat 1 tablespoon of the oil in a large skillet. Add the tempeh and stir over medium heat for 5 minutes. Transfer the tempeh to a bowl.

3. Heat the remaining tablespoon of oil in the pan. Add the garlic, carrots, pepper, and broccoli. Sauté over medium heat for 3 minutes. Add ½ cup of water, cover the pan, and simmer for 5 minutes, or until the vegetables are crisp-tender.

4. Return the tempeh to the pan, along with the scallions. Cook over medium heat for about 2 minutes, until everything is heated through. Serve with the peanut sauce.

MEDITERRANEAN CHICKPEAS

Chickpeas baked in a sauce of fresh tomatoes and garlic are a staple of Sicilian peasant cuisine. This is a superfast and easy version using canned tomatoes and frozen spinach. When you have more time, you can use fresh tomatoes and spinach for a more authentic flavor.

▶ **SERVES 6**

2 tablespoons extra virgin olive oil

1 cup coarsely chopped onion

3 garlic cloves, minced

Two 15-ounce cans chickpeas, drained and rinsed, or 3 cups cooked chickpeas

2 cups frozen chopped spinach, thawed and drained of all water

3 cups diced fresh tomatoes, or two 14-ounce cans

1 teaspoon red pepper flakes

1 teaspoon dried oregano

2 tablespoons fresh lemon juice

Salt and freshly ground black pepper

1. Heat the olive oil in a large skillet over medium heat. Add the onion and sauté for 5 minutes. Add the garlic and continue to sauté until the onion is just tender. Add the chickpeas, spinach, tomatoes, red pepper flakes, and oregano. Cover and simmer over low heat for 30 minutes. Remove from the heat and stir in the lemon juice. Add salt and black pepper to taste.

SWEET AND SPICY BAKED TOFU

Start this recipe at least 4 hours before you are ready to put it in the oven. Because tofu is porous and relatively bland, it absorbs flavors of marinades well. Hands-on preparation time is minimal, but pressing the tofu first and then letting it steep in the marinade for several hours will really enhance the flavor. The recipe calls for 14 ounces of tofu, but if your store sells tofu in 16-ounce packages, it's fine to use the whole thing—you don't need to adjust the other ingredients. Serve over rice, arrange over a bed of lettuce, or serve from a platter as an appetizer.

▶ SERVES 4

One 14-ounce package extra-firm tofu
¼ cup tamari
2 tablespoons pure maple syrup
1 tablespoon ketchup
1 tablespoon cider vinegar
Several drops hot pepper sauce, or to taste
¼ teaspoon garlic powder
¼ teaspoon black pepper
1 teaspoon liquid smoke

1. To press the tofu (if you don't have a tofu press), wrap in paper towels and place on a cookie sheet. Put a wooden cutting board on top and then place something heavy on top of that—a great big dictionary or a pot of water. Let sit for 30 minutes.

2. In a small bowl, combine the tamari, maple syrup, ketchup, vinegar, hot pepper sauce, garlic powder, pepper, and liquid smoke and set aside.

3. Remove the tofu from its press, and peel away the paper towels. Cut the tofu into ½-inch cubes and place in a casserole dish. Pour the marinade over the tofu, cover the dish, and marinate for at least 4 hours in the refrigerator.

4. Preheat the oven to 375°F. Bake the tofu for 30 minutes, turning it several times for even browning.

TRACY'S QUICK ENCHILADAS

These popular enchiladas (from Tracy Martin, who responded to the vegan survey Carol and Patti conducted in 2011) can be topped with vegan sour cream (such as Tofutti brand), salsa, avocados, or tomatoes. Once heated, cooled, and then reheated, these enchiladas are even better. Be sure to look for a canned green chile sauce that is vegan, since many brands contain pork. We recommend Hatch brand.

You may have a favorite kind of corn tortillas. We like to use the smaller-diameter tortillas; you will probably need twelve to fourteen tortillas for the layers.

▶ **SERVES 6 TO 8**

> Two 15-ounce cans vegan green chile sauce, such as Hatch brand
> 12 to 14 corn tortillas
> One 12-ounce bag frozen BOCA Crumbles, or Original Vegan
>   BOCA Burgers, crumbled
> One 16-ounce can refried beans
> One 15-ounce can whole black beans or pinto beans, drained and
>   rinsed
> 1 medium sweet onion, chopped
> One 10-ounce can chopped tomatoes with green chiles
> One 16-ounce bag frozen corn
> One 4.5-ounce can chopped green chiles, or some whole chiles
>   (if you can find fresh), roasted
> One 2.25-ounce can sliced black olives, optional
> 8 ounces meltable shredded vegan cheese, such as Daiya
>   Cheddar, optional

1. Preheat the oven to 350°F.
2. Pour the first can of green chile sauce into the bottom of a 9 × 13-inch baking dish. Cut or tear up the corn tortillas into quarters and spread half of them over the sauce.
3. Place half of the BOCA Crumbles into a separate bowl and stir

in the refried and whole beans, along with the chopped onion, tomatoes, and some of the frozen corn (about 1 cup). (Freeze the other half.)

4. Spread a layer of the mixture of Boca Crumbles and beans over the torn tortillas in the pan. Spread chopped or fresh roasted chiles on top. Add another layer of the torn pieces of tortilla.

5. Pour the other can of green chile sauce on top. Add the chopped black olives and/or vegan cheese, if using, to the top of the dish.

6. Bake until well heated and the tortilla edges are just a little crispy, about 25 minutes.

CORNY DOGS WITH A VEGAN FRYING BATTER

Every year people come to the Texas State Fair to discover something new that's being fried. As a Texan, the late Shirley Wilkes-Johnson saw one of her unique responsibilities to be the veganization of well-known Texas dishes, including those involving "frying batter." In addition to hot dogs, use this batter for onions, peppers, and—like those competitors at the State Fair—experiment!

▶ SERVES 8 TO 10

Oil for frying
8 to 10 vegan hot dogs
½ cup unbleached all-purpose flour
⅓ cup cornmeal
1 tablespoon nutritional yeast, optional
1½ teaspoons baking powder
½ teaspoon dry mustard
½ teaspoon salt
¼ teaspoon freshly ground white pepper
¼ teaspoon cayenne pepper (or to taste), optional
1 tablespoon Ener-G Egg Replacer
1 cup soy milk

1. Heat the oil in a deep fryer or electric skillet to 350°F.

2. Drain and dry the vegan hot dogs. Insert a Popsicle stick (see note) or wooden skewer into each, leaving enough of the stick on the outside to make a handle. Set aside.

3. Combine the flour and cornmeal in a large bowl and add the nutritional yeast, baking powder, mustard, salt, white pepper, and cayenne.

4. Combine 2 tablespoons of water and the egg replacer in a measuring cup and whisk until well mixed. Add the soy milk and whisk until well mixed. Whisk this into the flour mixture.

5. Dip the hot dogs into the batter to coat. Immerse them in the hot oil and fry until golden and crispy. Drain on paper towels. Serve hot.

NOTE: You can buy Popsicle sticks at any craft or teacher supply store, or even a dollar store.

NEATLOAF

This recipe, an adaptation of the continual, hands-down meat eater's favorite, is from Jennifer Raymond's book *The Peaceful Palate*. Sliced leftovers make great sandwiches. Some cooks adapt the recipe by adding a little tomato paste to the mix. Jennifer puts ketchup over the top. Try it both ways and see which way you like it.

Jennifer justifiably recommends using a food processor; it quickly makes each ingredient the right size for mixing together. Once you have whizzed the oats in your food processor, it is very easy to use it to chop up the mushrooms, bell pepper, and carrot, using the same blade.

▶ **SERVES 8**

1 cup uncooked quick-cooking rolled oats

2 cups cooked brown rice

1 cup wheat germ

1 cup finely chopped walnuts or sunflower seeds

1 cup chopped mushrooms

1 onion, finely chopped

½ medium bell pepper, seeded and finely chopped

1 medium carrot, shredded or finely chopped

½ teaspoon dried thyme

½ teaspoon dried marjoram

1 teaspoon dried sage

2 tablespoons soy sauce

2 tablespoons stone-ground or Dijon mustard

1 tablespoon peanut butter

5 tablespoons vegan ketchup or BBQ Sauce, or 3 tablespoons
    tomato paste

1. Preheat the oven to 350°F. Grease a 9 × 5-inch loaf pan.

2. Whiz the rolled oats in a dry food processor. Transfer to a bowl.

3. Add all the remaining ingredients, except the ketchup or BBQ Sauce, to the oats and mix for 2 minutes with a large spoon. This will help to bind the loaf together.

4. Pat the ingredients into the prepared pan and top with the ketchup. Bake until lightly browned, or about 1 hour. Let stand for 10 minutes before serving.

TURKEY'S FAVORITE BREAD DRESSING

Adapted from Jennifer Raymond's *The Peaceful Palate,* this "stuffing" will bring the taste of Thanksgiving to your table any time of year. Serve it with Mashed Potatoes and Gravy (page 285) and Cranberry Fig Relish (page 254) for a trio of traditional holiday flavors.

▶ SERVES 8

1 tablespoon extra virgin olive oil

1 onion, chopped

3 cups sliced mushrooms (about ½ pound)

2 celery stalks, sliced

4 cups cubed bread

⅓ cup finely chopped fresh parsley

⅓ cup fresh thyme

½ teaspoon dried marjoram

½ teaspoon dried sage

⅛ teaspoon freshly ground black pepper

½ teaspoon salt

About 1 cup very hot water or vegan vegetable stock

1. Preheat the oven to 350°F. Spray a 9 × 13-inch baking dish with cooking oil spray.

2. Heat the oil in a large pot or skillet and sauté the onion for 5 minutes. Add the mushrooms and celery and cook over medium heat until the mushrooms begin to brown, about 5 minutes.

3. Stir in the bread, parsley, thyme, marjoram, sage, black pepper, and salt. Lower the heat and continue to cook for 3 minutes. Stir in the water or stock, a little at a time, until the dressing obtains desired moistness.

4. Spread the dressing in the prepared baking dish, cover, and bake for 20 minutes. Remove the cover and bake for 10 minutes longer.

SHIRLEY'S MOUSSAKA

Even people who think they don't like eggplant will be surprised when they like this recipe—Shirley Wilkes-Johnson's vegan version of a traditional Greek dish. It calls for veggie ground beef but that can be left out. While potatoes are not usually in traditional moussaka, they make it even better. You can use zucchini instead of, or in addition to, potatoes. If you don't have a Vitamix or other high-powered blender, soak the cashews for at least an hour or up to overnight before blending.

Any leftovers will be even more delicious the next day.

▶ SERVES 8

Salt

3 medium to large eggplants, stem ends trimmed, sliced
lengthwise into ½-inch slices

6 to 8 medium potatoes, peeled and sliced into ½-inch slices

1 tablespoon extra virgin olive oil, plus more for brushing the
vegetables

1 cup chopped onion

1 medium-size red bell pepper, seeded and chopped

One 8-ounce package mushrooms, chopped or quartered

One 14.5-ounce can diced tomatoes

2 tablespoons tomato paste

One 12-ounce package ground beef–style veggie meat (such as
BOCA Ground Crumbles or Yves or Lightlife brand), optional

¼ cup chopped fresh parsley

1 teaspoon ground cumin

½ teaspoon freshly ground black pepper

¼ teaspoon ground cinnamon

¼ teaspoon freshly grated nutmeg

Béchamel Sauce:

½ cup raw cashews

2½ cups water

2 tablespoons cornstarch

1 teaspoon onion powder

¾ teaspoon salt

¼ teaspoon white pepper

1. Sprinkle salt on the eggplant slices. Place them in a colander and allow them to sit for 30 minutes to 1 hour. Rinse and pat dry. (You may omit this step entirely, if desired.)

2. Preheat the oven to 400°F and spray 2 baking sheets with cooking oil spray.

3. Place the eggplant and potato slices on the prepared baking sheets and brush them with oil. Bake for 20 to 25 minutes. Lower the oven temperature to 350°F.

4. Meanwhile, heat the olive oil in a large skillet. Add the onion, bell pepper, and mushrooms and sauté over medium-high heat for about 5 minutes. Stir in the tomatoes and tomato paste until mixed. Add the veggie meat, parsley, cumin, pepper, cinnamon, nutmeg, and salt to taste.

5. Spray the bottom of a 13 × 9-inch baking pan with nonstick spray. Place a layer of eggplant slices in the pan and then a layer of potato slices. Add the veggie meat mixture, cover with the remaining potato slices, and then the remaining eggplant slices.

6. To prepare the sauce, blend all the ingredients together in a blender. Transfer to a medium sauce pan and bring to a low boil, stirring constantly until the mixture thickens. Pour the sauce over the eggplant.

7. Bake at 350°F for 30 to 35 minutes. Allow to cool for 10 minutes before serving.

STUFFED SEITAN ROAST

Seitan, or "wheat meat," is easy to make. We've given you Sandy Weiland's favorite recipe on page 231, and Eddy Garza's BBQ seitan sandwich on page 277. But for an impressive dinner entrée, choose this recipe. Served on your favorite platter, its appearance alone may elicit delight. Then the excitement continues as everyone bites in.

Carol adapted the roast, stuffed with spinach, mushrooms, and pine nuts, from her friend Molly Kirby's recipe.

▶ **SERVES 8**

Seitan Roast:
 2 cups gluten powder (vital wheat gluten)
 ¼ cup nutritional yeast
 2 tablespoons barley flour
 1 teaspoon ground cumin

1 teaspoon ground coriander

½ teaspoon garlic powder

¼ cup fresh basil, minced

2 tablespoons vegan BBQ sauce (see recipe on page 277 or
   purchase the sauce of your choice)

1¼ cups vegan vegetable stock or broth

2 tablespoons tamari

1 tablespoon olive oil

1 tablespoon cider vinegar

Filling:

One 8-ounce container vegan cream cheese

2 cups spinach

1½ pounds shiitake or oyster mushrooms, sliced and roasted in a
   425°F oven for 10 minutes

½ cup pine nuts

Broth:

1¾ cups vegan vegetable stock or broth

¼ cup red wine

3 garlic cloves, diced

1 tablespoon tamari

Fresh rosemary for garnish

1. To prepare the seitan: Combine the gluten powder, nutritional yeast, barley flour, cumin, coriander, garlic powder, and basil in a large bowl. Form a well in the mixture.

2. In a measuring cup or small bowl, stir together the BBQ sauce, vegetable stock, tamari, oil, and vinegar. Pour into the well of the vital wheat gluten mixture. Stir to combine until the gluten mixture is completely moistened. Knead the seitan for 5 minutes.

3. Heat the oven to 375°F. Oil a 13 × 9-inch baking dish. Place the seitan mixture on parchment paper, plastic wrap, or wax paper. Cover with plastic wrap and use a rolling pin to roll out into a roughly 13 × 9-inch rectangle.

4. To fill the seitan, spread the cream cheese on the rectangle, leaving a 1-inch margin along the sides. Arrange the spinach and roasted mushrooms on top of the cream cheese. Sprinkle with the pine nuts.
5. Roll up the seitan jelly-roll style. Tightly pinch together the ends. Create a seam by pinching the seitan together along the length of the roll to completely seal the ingredients inside. (Do not allow any stuffing to leak.)
6. Carefully transfer the roll to the prepared baking dish, seam side down.
7. In a measuring cup, prepare the broth: Mix the vegetable stock, wine, garlic, and tamari. Pour over the seitan and add a few sprigs of fresh rosemary. Seal the baking dish with foil.
8. Bake for 30 minutes. Carefully flip over the seitan roll. Baste the top with some of the broth from the pan, re-cover with foil, and bake for about 30 minutes more.

TWO VARIATIONS

Seitan with Roasted Vegetables

Add vegetables, such as zucchini, yellow squash, parsnip, turnip, carrots, and potatoes. Cut the vegetables into bite-size pieces, arrange them around the seitan, and let them roast while the seitan cooks.

Seitan en Croûte

For this variation, you will need a box of vegan puff pastry, such as from Pepperidge Farm.

Assemble and cook the seitan a couple of days before you plan to serve it. Allow it to cool overnight in the refrigerator, or freeze it. (On the day you are going to serve it, remove it from the freezer in the morning.) Twenty minutes before you want to bake it, defrost the puff pastry according to the directions on the package.

Place one sheet of the puff pastry on a baking dish or casserole and pull or stretch the sheet to accommodate the size of the seitan roll. Place the seitan roll on top. Use the second pastry sheet to completely cover the seitan roll. Stretch both of the pastry sheets so their edges meet. Join the edges of the sheets together and apply a little water to seal them completely.

Bake in a preheated 400°F oven for 20 minutes, or until the pastry is puffed up and golden.

DESSERTS

Vegans eat dessert just like everyone else. It's surprisingly easy to create both decadent treats and healthier choices without eggs or dairy foods. Using the tips we shared in chapter 10, you'll find that you can adapt most of your old family favorites to make them vegan. In this section we share some of the recipes that we and other vegans have had great success with—whether it's for a special occasion or one of those times when you just need something sweet.

ZUCCHINI BREAD

A dessert bread that can be toasted, eaten for breakfast, or served with afternoon coffee or tea is an excellent way to get everyone eating zucchini. You can double the recipe and give the second loaf to a friend, or freeze it for later. This recipe is another creation of Shirley Wilkes-Johnson.

▶ MAKES 1 LOAF; SERVES 12

2 cups unbleached all-purpose flour
¾ cup organic sugar (see box on page 228)
1 tablespoon nutritional yeast
1 teaspoon ground cinnamon
1 teaspoon baking powder
½ teaspoon baking soda
¼ teaspoon salt
¼ teaspoon freshly grated nutmeg

1 cup loosely packed shredded unpeeled zucchini

⅔ cup soy milk

¼ cup soy or canola oil

1 teaspoon grated lemon zest

2 tablespoons fresh lemon juice

½ cup coarsely chopped walnuts

1. Preheat the oven to 325°F.

2. Stir together the flour, sugar, nutritional yeast, cinnamon, baking powder, baking soda, salt, and nutmeg in a medium mixing bowl. Set aside.

3. Mix together the zucchini, soy milk, oil, lemon zest, and lemon juice, in a separate bowl. Stir the wet and dry mixtures together; do not overmix. The batter consistency should be thick. Stir in the walnuts.

4. Coat a 9 × 5 × 3-inch loaf pan with nonstick cooking oil spray. Pour the batter into the pan and bake on the middle rack of the oven for about 55 minutes, or until a toothpick inserted into the center of the loaf comes out clean.

5. Let the bread cool in the pan for 10 minutes, then transfer to a wire rack to finish cooling.

MOM'S VEGAN CINNAMON ROLLS

Christina Nakhoda (page 226) veganized her family's traditional cinnamon rolls, to the joy of her family and friends. Christina likes to make her rolls very "cinnamon-y," so this recipe calls for more cinnamon in the filling than you might find in traditional recipes. You can use less if you prefer.

▶ MAKES 12 ROLLS

1 tablespoon instant or quick active dry yeast

¼ cup warm water (110°F)

1¼ cups soy milk, heated for about 1 minute in the microwave or
    3 minutes on the stove and then cooled to room temperature

8 tablespoons (1 stick) vegan margarine, at room temperature

Ener-G Egg Replacer to equal 3 eggs

1 teaspoon salt

1½ cups granulated sugar

5 cups all-purpose unbleached bread flour, or more as needed

¼ cup ground cinnamon

8 tablespoons (1 stick) vegan margarine, melted

Vanilla Frosting:

1 pound confectioners' sugar (4½ cups)

½ teaspoon pure almond extract

2 tablespoons plant-based milk, such as almond, soy, or coconut,
plus more if needed

1. Soften the yeast in the warm water. Let the yeast activate 3 to 5 minutes, until foamy.

2. In the large bowl of a standing electric mixer, mix the yeast mixture, soy milk, margarine, prepared egg replacer, salt, and ¾ cup of the granulated sugar. Stir to ensure it is all combined. Add the flour and beat with dough hook until a soft dough forms (see note).

3. Remove the dough from the mixer and knead for 2 to 3 minutes on a floured surface. Place the dough in a well-oiled bowl. Cover and let rise until doubled in size, or cover and place in refrigerator up to 5 days.

4. Preheat the oven to 350°F. Oil a 13 × 9 × 2-inch baking pan; set aside. Combine the remaining ¾ cup of granulated sugar and all of the cinnamon in a small bowl and set aside.

5. After the dough has risen, place on a floured surface; using a rolling pin, roll out to roughly a 25 × 16-inch rectangle. Brush the melted margarine over the top of the dough and sprinkle generously with the cinnamon-sugar mixture.

6. Starting on a long edge, roll up jelly-roll fashion; pinch the seams to seal. Cut into twelve slices and place each slice cut side down in the prepared pan. Cover and let rise in a warm place until doubled in size—45 minutes to 1 hour.

7. Bake for about 20 minutes, or until the rolls are light golden brown.

8. Let cool 5 minutes in the pan.

9. While the rolls bake, prepare the frosting: Stir or beat the frosting ingredients with a hand mixer at medium speed, adding more milk 1 teaspoon at a time, until the frosting is smooth and a spreadable consistency. Frost the warm rolls while they are still in the pan.

NOTE: The dough should form an elastic ball, not too sticky. If you think the dough is too moist, add additional flour 1 tablespoon at a time. If you think the dough is looking too dry and not smooth, add water 1 tablespoon at a time. It should be just slightly tacky to the touch.

VARIATIONS

- Top the frosting with finely chopped pecans or walnuts.
- Arrange raisins on the top of cinnamon-sugar filling before rolling up.
- After rolling out the dough into a rectangle, spread the dough with mixture of 8 tablespoons (1 stick) of vegan margarine, melted, ½ cup of granulated sugar, and 1 tablespoon of freshly grated orange zest.
- Use an alternative cinnamon filling made with 1 cup soft brown sugar mixed with 5 tablespoons ground cinnamon.

MARZIPAN AND STRAWBERRIES DIPPED IN CHOCOLATE

Every year for Passover, Patti's husband dips marzipan and strawberries into melted chocolate for dessert. This family tradition never fails to elicit cheers, especially from guests with a sweet tooth.

▶ SERVES 8 TO 10

12 large strawberries, plus more for serving plain, or undipped

One 7-ounce tube marzipan (available in the baking section of
most supermarkets)
One 8- or 9-ounce bag vegan chocolate chips (see note about
chocolate on page 163)
1 tablespoon canola oil (to prevent the chocolate from hardening
too quickly), optional

1. Line a baking sheet with parchment paper. Wash and thoroughly
dry the strawberries. Slice the marzipan into rounds about ¼ inch
thick.

2. Combine the chips and oil (if using) in a glass bowl or measuring
cup and melt in a microwave oven: Heat for 30 seconds, stir, and, if
needed, heat for another 30 seconds. Continue stirring until all the
chips are melted. (This may require one more 15-second heating in
the microwave.) Alternatively, you can melt them in a double boiler
on the stove, stirring over medium heat until completely melted.

3. Using a fork, dip each strawberry into the chocolate, then place
each strawberry on the lined baking sheet. Again using a fork, dip
each marzipan circle into the chocolate, and then place each circle on
the lined baking sheet. Refrigerate the filled baking sheet for at least
1 hour, or until ready to serve.

HUMMINGBIRD CAKE

There doesn't seem to be an agreed upon explanation for the unique and
whimsical name given to this delightfully sweet cake. It achieved mass appeal
after appearing in the February 1978 issue of *Southern Living Magazine* and
for many years "Hummingbird Cake" was the publication's most requested
recipe. In addition to making this family favorite vegan-friendly, Carol's friend
Christina Nakhoda further modified it by adding coconut and some extra
spices not called for in the original recipe. Hummingbird Cake stays fresh in
the refrigerator for days, or it can be frozen and served weeks later.

▶ MAKES ONE 9-INCH 3-LAYER CAKE; SERVES 12

3 cups all-purpose flour

1 cup granulated sugar

½ cup turbinado sugar

1 tablespoon Ener-G Egg Replacer

1 teaspoon baking soda

1 teaspoon salt

1 teaspoon ground cinnamon

1 teaspoon ground ginger

1 teaspoon freshly grated nutmeg

1 cup applesauce

One 8-ounce can crushed pineapple in juice, undrained

2 to 3 ripe bananas, mashed (about 1½ cups)

¾ cup vegetable oil

½ cup fresh orange juice

2 teaspoon pure vanilla extract

1 cup finely chopped pecans

1 cup sweetened shredded coconut

Cream Cheese Frosting:

One 8-ounce container vegan cream cheese

8 tablespoons (1 stick) vegan margarine, at room temperature

2 pounds confectioners' sugar (about 9 cups)

1 teaspoon pure vanilla extract

Plant-based milk such as soy, almond, or coconut, as needed

1 cup chopped pecans, or 16 pecan halves for garnish, optional

1. Preheat the oven to 350°F. Grease three 9-inch round cake pans.
2. In a large mixing bowl, place all the dry ingredients and mix thoroughly. Add the applesauce, pineapple, bananas, oil, orange juice, vanilla extract, pecans, and coconut. Stir until combined; do not beat.
3. Divide batter evenly among the prepared cake pans. Bake for 25 to 30 minutes until a toothpick inserted near the center comes out clean. Cool pans on a wire rack.

4. Prepare the frosting: In the bowl of a standing electric mixer (or with a hand mixer), beat the cream cheese, margarine, and confectioners' sugar until smooth.

5. Beat in the vanilla and enough milk to make a frosting of the desired consistency.

6. When the cake is completely cool, frost using ¾ cup of frosting on each layer and the remaining frosting on the sides and top of cake.

7. If desired, use the optional chopped pecans to decorate the sides or the top layer of the cake; or, arrange sixteen pecan halves on top of the frosted cake.

TEXAS CHOCOLATE SHEET CAKE

Shirley Wilkes-Johnson called this "a rather decadent, old-fashioned recipe." Use a jelly-roll pan to achieve just the right thickness in the cake. A jelly-roll pan is about 15 × 10 inches with 1-inch sides. It's similar to a large cookie sheet. You can use a 13 × 9-inch baking pan, but the cake will be thicker. One summer, Carol made three of these cakes for a family celebration. *Everyone* loved the cake—even those who didn't think they would.

▶ **MAKES ONE 15 X 10–INCH CAKE; SERVES 35 (2-INCH SQUARE PIECES)**

1 cup soy milk
1 tablespoon cider vinegar
2 cups all-purpose flour
2 cups organic sugar (see box on page 228)
1 teaspoon baking soda
½ pound (2 sticks) vegan margarine, at room temperature
⅓ cup unsweetened cocoa powder
2 teaspoons pure vanilla extract

Chocolate Pecan Icing:
8 tablespoons (1 stick) vegan margarine, at room temperature

¼ cup unsweetened cocoa powder, sifted

1 pound confectioners' sugar (about 4½ cups)

⅓ cup soy milk

1 teaspoon pure vanilla extract

1 cup chopped pecans

1. Preheat the oven to 375°F. Grease a 15 × 10-inch jelly-roll pan. Combine the soy milk and cider vinegar in a mixing cup, and set aside.

2. Combine the flour, sugar, and baking soda in a medium bowl. Mix well and set aside.

3. Mix together the margarine, cocoa powder, and 1 cup of water in a medium saucepan. Heat to boiling over medium heat, while stirring often. Pour over the flour and sugar mixture. Add the vanilla to the soy milk and vinegar mixture, and then whisk into the other ingredients. Turn the batter into the prepared pan.

4. Bake for 20 to 25 minutes, or until a toothpick inserted into the center comes out clean.

5. While the cake bakes, prepare the icing: Combine the margarine, cocoa powder, and soy milk in a medium bowl and beat with an electric mixer on medium speed for about 2 minutes, until light and fluffy. Add the confectioners' sugar and vanilla and beat on high speed until well mixed. Stir in the pecans.

6. Immediately frost the top of the hot cake with the Chocolate Pecan Icing. (Don't let the cake cool before frosting.) Allow the cake to cool, and then cut it into squares.

BANANA CAKE

Because she considers this a foolproof recipe, Patti prepares it for celebrations throughout the year. Serve it with vegan ice cream. It's another winner from Jennifer Raymond.

▶ **MAKES ONE 9-INCH SQUARE CAKE; SERVES 9**

2 cups unbleached or whole wheat pastry flour
1½ teaspoons baking soda
½ teaspoon salt
1 cup sugar or other sweetener
⅓ cup canola or safflower oil
4 ripe bananas, mashed (about 2½ cups)
1 teaspoon pure vanilla extract
1 cup chopped walnuts, optional
½ cup vegan chocolate chips, optional

1. Preheat the oven to 350°F. Spray a 9-inch square baking pan with cooking oil spray.
2. Mix the flour, baking soda, and salt together.
3. Beat the sugar and oil together in a large bowl. Add the mashed bananas. Stir in ¼ cup of water and the vanilla and mix thoroughly. Add the flour mixture, along with the chopped walnuts and chocolate chips, if using, and stir to mix. Spread into the prepared pan, and bake for about 45 to 50 minutes, or until a toothpick inserted into the center comes out clean.

PERMISSIONS ACKNOWLEDGMENTS

Grateful acknowledgment is made for permission to include (and in some cases to reprint) the following material:

- Jasmin Singer and Mariann Sullivan of OurHenHouse.org for permission to use the story of Jasmin's grandmother, Sherrey Reim Glickman that first appeared on their website.
- Karol Crosbie, for permission to reprint "The Vegan Potluck" on page 170, which appeared in the Spring 2013 issue of *Wooster* magazine, Karol Crosbie, editor.
- Monica Cohen, Heather Fliehman, and the Vegetarian Resource Group (vrg.org), for permission to reprint the Protein/Calorie Drink on page 198.
- VegWeb.com and Colleen Holland for permission to reprint Dragonfly's Bulk, Dry Uncheese Mix on page 224.
- Bryanna Clark Grogan, for permission to reprint the Vegan Mayo recipe on page 228.
- Sandy Weiland, for permission to reprint the Vegan Sausage recipe on page 231.
- Brenda Davis, for permission to reprint the Up from Oatmeal recipe on page 243.
- Rae Sikora, for permission to reprint the Crock Cheese recipe on page 248.
- Miyoko Schinner for permission to reprint the Very Benevolent Caesar Dressing recipe on page 257.
- The George Mateljan Foundation, for permission to reprint the Carrot Coconut Soup recipe on page 270.

- Eddie Garza, for permission to reprint the BBQ "Beef" Sandwiches with Beef-Style Seitan recipe on page 277.
- Jennifer Raymond, for permission to reprint Mashed Potatoes and Gravy (page 285), Neatloaf (page 310), Turkey's Favorite Bread Dressing (page 311), and Banana Cake (page 325).
- JL Fields, for permission to reprint White Bean Gravy with Ginger and Cinnamon on page 286 and Almond-Miso Sauce on page 296.
- The Dallas-based Vegetarian Education Network for permission to reprint Spice Options for Grains and Legumes on pages 290–294.
- Christina Nakhoda, for permission to reprint Black-Bean Burgers with Mango BBQ Sauce on page 297, Cinnamon Rolls on page 318, and Hummingbird Cake on page 321.
- The Experiment, LLC, for permission to reprint the "Mango BBQ Sauce" recipe, page 298, adapted from *Veggie Burgers Every Which Way* by Lukas Volger, Copyright © Lukas Volger, 2010.
- Colleen Welsh, for permission to reprint Beans and Greens on page 299 and "Chicken" Piccata on page 301.
- Helen R. Moy, for permission to reprint the Mac and Cheese recipe on page 302.
- Lantern Press, for permission to reprint the Lasagna recipe on page 303 from *How to Eat Like a Vegetarian Even If You Never Want to Be One*, by Carol J. Adams and Patti Breitman. Copyright © Carol J. Adams and Patti Breitman, 2008.
- Tracy Martin, for permission to reprint Tracy's Quick Enchiladas on page 308.
- Ben Johnson, for permission to use the following recipes developed by the late Shirley Wilkes-Johnson: Zucchini Bread (page 317), Sweet and Sour Red Cabbage (page 284), Feta/Cottage Cheese (page 222), Shirley's Moussaka (page 312), Corny Dogs (page 309), Confetti Slaw (page 258), Cajun-Style Eggless Salad (page 261), Southwestern Corn Salad (page 266), and Texas Chocolate Sheet Cake (page 323).

ACKNOWLEDGMENTS

From Carol, Patti, and Ginny: Thank you to our publisher and editor Matthew Lore for his great enthusiasm for this book and for guiding us with wisdom, warmth, and careful editing through its production. And to the whole brilliant team at The Experiment: Associate Publisher Dan O'Connor, publicists Jack Palmer and Sarah Schneider, designers Pauline Neuwirth and Christine Van Bree, copy editor Iris Bass, proofreader Deri Reed, and indexer Wendy Allex, for their expert help in creating and promoting this book.

We're indebted to Patti's friend David Hoffman for giving us our book title and to Christine Moen, who spent many hours organizing and revising the first draft of our recipes.

When Ginny requested stories from her blog readers who had gone vegan after the age of fifty, she received well over a hundred replies. Thank you to everyone who took the time to respond and also to those who answered the survey on "what vegans eat" that Carol and Patti conducted in 2011. Many of the responses to both of these requests are included in this book.

Thank you, too, to those who generously shared recipes with us: Jennifer Raymond, Miyoko Schinner, The George Mateljan Foundation's World's Healthiest Foods, Colleen Holland, JL Fields, Brenda Davis, Helen R. Moy, Sandy Weiland, Eddie Garza, Monica Cohen, Bryanna Clark Grogran, Heather Fliehman and the Vegetarian Resource Group, Rae Sikora, Colleen Welsh, Christina Nakhoda, Tracy Martin, and Ben Johnson on behalf of his late wife Shirley Wilkes-Johnson.

Thank you to those who agreed to allow our interviews with them to become stories in this book: Colleen Welsh, Sam Kelly, Marc Bekoff,

Greg Shaurette, Marisa Monagle, Sandy Weiland, Donald Moy, Roni Omohundro, and Christina Nakhoda.

We are thankful for Charles Stahler of the Vegetarian Resource Group and Dr. Neal Barnard of Physicians Committee for Responsible Medicine who were of great help in answering questions about serving the needs of vegans in retirement facilities.

Kim Sturla of Animal Place was generous with her firsthand information about farmed animals. We thank lauren Ornelas and The Food Empowerment Project, for bringing a focus to food justice and information about chocolate; and Dr. Michael Greger of nutritionfacts.org.

From Carol: I thank Bruce Buchanan for thirty-five years of supporting my writing career and my exploration of plant-based food and recipes. I am also thankful that because of my sisters, Nancy Adams and Jane Adams, we together were able to provide caregiving for our parents in their home until the day they died—and during those years, we sisters shared not only caregiving, but care for each other, including vegan food for me. What a difference that made!

I also thank Jennifer Zdunczyk, Director of Dining Services at Medford Leas, Medford, NJ, and Godwin Dixon of Presbyterian Communities Services for discussing vegan food in nursing homes with me. Lori Gruen and Josephine Donovan were early supporters of this project.

From Patti: I send abundant thanks to my mom, Fran Zitner, for a lifetime of unwavering love and support. And to my husband, Stan Rosenfeld, for being a stalwart and kind recipe taster and a mensch of the first order.

I also thank Farm Sanctuary, Mercy for Animals, especially for their *Vegetarian Starter Kit*, Karen Davis and United Poultry Concerns, Pamela Rice and *101 Reasons Why I'm a Vegetarian*, and Meredith McCarty and Healing Cuisine. And gratitude to Dominique Blanchard for years of invaluable assistance and inspiration at my cooking classes.

From Ginny: I'm grateful to know and work with so many nutrition experts who advocate for animals and for healthy vegan diets. Jack Norris, RD, and Reed Mangels, PhD, RD, remain my go-to experts on vegan nutrition. Thank you, also, to my brilliant colleagues Brenda Davis, RD; Vesanto Melina, MS, RD; Matt Ruscigno, MPH, RD; Mark Rifkin, MS, RD; Carolyn Tampe, MS, RD; Ed Coffin; RD, Paul Appleby; and Stephen Walsh.

I'm fortunate to know so many wonderful activists who approach their work with a heart for animals and a commitment to scientific integrity. Thank you to Matt Ball and Anne Green of Vegan Outreach; David Sutherland and Debra Stephens of Vegan Chicago; Unny Nambudiripad and Dave Rolsky of Compassionate Action for Animals.

Love and gratitude to my best vegan buddies JL Fields, Erik Marcus, Louise Holton, Lisa Herzstein, Phyllis Becker, and Kate Schumann.

I am grateful to my brothers and their families for their love and support. My parents Willie Schrenk Kisch and Bill Kisch remain sources of support and strength even though temporarily gone from my sight.

And as always, I am blessed to be married to Mark Messina, nutrition advisor, recipe taste tester, animal advocate, and world's best husband.

NOTES

CHAPTER 3. WHY VEGAN?

1. *Livestock's Long Shadow: Environmental Issues and Options* Rome: Food and Agriculture Organization of the United Nations, 2006, chapter 4.5, p. 167. ftp://ftp.fao.org/docrep/fao/010/a0701e/a0701e.pdf
2. Livestock's Long Shadow, chapter 4.3.1, p. 136.
3. *Manure Use for Fertilizer and for Energy / Report to Congress.* Washington: United States Department of Agriculture, p. 4 http://ers.usda.gov/media/377381/ap037a_1_.pdf.
4. *Manure Use for Fertilizer and for Energy / Report to Congress,* p. 5
5. World Food Programme, Hunger Statistics, http://www.wfp.org/hunger/stats.
6. Walden Bello, "Cows Eat Better Than People Do," published by Beyond Beef, 1992, posted to the web at http://unreasonable.org/wrapper/vegan/BeyondBeefBello.html
7. United States Department of Census, "World Population: 1950–2050." http://www.census.gov/population/international/data/idb/worldpopgraph.php
8. Mary Midgley, *Animals and Why They Matter.* Athens: University of Geogia Press, 1983, p. 27.
9. "Employee Describes Deliberate Torture of Chickens at Tyson Slaughter Plant." From the affidavit testimony of Virgil Butler, January 30, 2003. Reprinted in *Poultry Press,* publication of United Poultry Concerns, vol. 13, no. 1, Spring 2003. http://www.upc-online.org/spring03/tysons.htm
10. From an interview in *Friends of Hilda* newsletter 10, no. 1, published by Farm Sanctuary, Farm Sanctuary National Headquarters, P.O. Box 150, Watkins Glen, NY 14891

CHAPTER 4. WHY AND HOW WE AGE

1. H. Takata et al., "Influence of Major Histocompatibility Complex Region Genes on Human Longevity Among Okinawan-Japanese Centenarians and Nonagenarians," *The Lancet* 3, no. 8563 (October 10 1987): 824–26.
2. L. Hayflick, "The Limited in Vitro Lifetime of Human Diploid Cell Strains," *Experimental Cell Research* 37 (March 1965): 614–36.
3. D. Ornish, et al. "Increased Telomerase Activity and Comprehensive Lifestyle Changes: A Pilot Study," *The Lancet Oncology* 9, no. 11 (November 2008): 1048–57.
4. G. Sartorius, et al., "Serum Testosterone, Dihydrotestosterone and Estradiol Concentrations in Older Men Self-Reporting Very Good Health: The Healthy Man Study," *Clinical Endocrinology (Oxford).* 77, no. 5 (November 2012): 755–63.
5. F. C. Bennett and D. M. Ingram, "Diet and Female Sex Hormone Concentrations: An Intervention Study for the Type of Fat Consumed," *American Journal of Clinical Nutrition* 52, no. 5 (1990): 808–12; M. Aubertin-Leheudre et al., "Diets and Hormonal Levels in Postmenopausal

Women with or Without Breast Cancer," *Nutrition and Cancer* 63, no. 4 (2011): 514–24; T. D. Shultz and N. E. Leklem, "Nutrient Intake and Hormonal Status of Premenopausal Vegetarian Seventh-Day Adventists and Premenopausal Nonvegetarians," *Nutrition and Cancer* 4, no. 4 (1983): 247–59.

6. K. Taku et al., "Extracted or Synthesized Soybean Isoflavones Reduce Menopausal Hot Flash Frequency and Severity: Systematic Review and Meta-Analysis of Randomized Controlled Trials," *Menopause* 19, no. 7 (July 2012): 776–90.

7. P. S. Williamson-Hughes et al., "Isoflavone Supplements Containing Predominantly Genistein Reduce Hot Flash Symptoms: A Critical Review of Published Studies," *Menopause* 13, no. 5 (September–October 2006): 831–39.

8. J. M. Hamilton-Reeves et al., "Clinical Studies Show No Effects of Soy Protein or Isoflavones on Reproductive Hormones In Men: Results of a Meta-Analysis," *Fertility and Sterility* 94, no. 3 (June 11, 2009): 997–1007.

9. J. H. Mitchell et al., " Effect of a Phytoestrogen Food Supplement on Reproductive Health in Normal Males, *Clinical Science (London)* 100, no. 6 (June 2001): 613–18.

10. M. Messina et al., "Report on the 8th International Symposium on the Role of Soy in Health Promotion and Chronic Disease Prevention and Treatment," *Journal of Nutrition* 139, no. 4 (April 2009): 796S–802S.

11. M. Messina, et al., "Estimated Asian Adult Soy Protein and Isoflavone Intakes," *Nutrition and Cancer* 55, no. 1 (2006): 1–12.

12. G. L. Grove and A. M. Kligman, "Age-Associated Changes in Human Epidermal Cell Renewal," *Journal of Gerontolology* 38, no. 2 (March 1983): 137–42.

13. A. M. Fjell and K. B. Walhovd. "Structural Brain Changes in Aging: Courses, Causes and Cognitive Consequences," *Reviews in the Neurosciences* 21, no. 3 (2010): 187–221.

CHAPTER 5. A HEALTHY DIET FOR 50+ VEGANS

1. E. E. Devore, et al., "Dietary Intakes of Berries and Flavonoids in Relation to Cognitive Decline," *Annals of Neurology* 72, no. 1 (July 20121): 135–43.

2. J. Lee et al., "Carotenoid Supplementation Reduces Erythema in Human Skin After Simulated Solar Radiation Exposure," *Proceedings of the Society for Experimental Biolology and Medicine* 22, no. 2 (February 2000): 170–74; W. Stahl et al., "Lycopene-rich Products and Dietary Photoprotection," *Photochemical and Photobiological Sciiences* 5, no. 2 (February 2006: 238–42; W. Stahl et al., "Dietary Tomato Paste Protects Against Ultraviolet Light-Induced Erythema in Humans," *Journal of Nutrition* 131, no. 5 (May 2001): 1449–51.

3. P. N. Appleby et al., "Diet, Vegetarianism, and Cataract Risk," *American Journal of Clinical Nutrition* 93, no. 5 (May 2011): 1128–35.

4. S. J. Hodges et al., "Circulating Levels of Vitamins K1 and K2 Decreased in Elderly Women with Hip Fracture," *Journal of Bone and Mineral Research* 8, no. 10 (October 1993): 1241–45; D. Feskanich et al., "Vitamin K Intake and Hip Fractures in Women: A Prospective Study," *American Journal of Clinical Nutrition* 69, no. 1 (1999): 74–79; S. L. Booth et al., "Vitamin K Intake and Bone Mineral Density in Women and Men," *American Journal of Clinical Nutrition* 77, no. 2 (February 2003): 512–16.

5. C. J. Prynne et al., "Fruit and Vegetable Intakes and Bone Mineral Status: A Cross Sectional Study in 5 Age and Sex Cohorts," *American Journal of Clinical Nutrition* 83, no. 6 (June 2006): 1420–28.

6. T. A. Sanders, "DHA Status of Vegetarians," *Prostaglandins Leukotrienes and Essential Fatty Acids* 8, no. 2–3 (August–September 2009): 137–41.

7. M. C. Morris, et al., "Consumption of Fish and n-3 Fatty Acids and Risk of Incident Alzheimer Disease," *Archives of Neurolology* 60, no. 7 (July 2003): 940–46; E. J. Schaefer et al., "Plasma Phosphatidylcholine Docosahexaenoic Acid Content and Risk of Dementia and Alzheimer Disease: The Framingham Heart Study," *Archives of Neurology* 63, no. 11 (November 2006): 1545–50.

8. P. Y. Lin and K. P. Su, "A Meta-Analytic Review of Double-Blind, Placebo-Controlled Trials of Antidepressant Efficacy of Omega-3 Fatty Acids," *Journal of Clinical Psychiatry* 68, no. 7 (July 2007): 1056–61; J. Sontrop and M. K. Campbell "Omega-3 Polyunsaturated Fatty Acids and Depression: A Review of the Evidence and a Methodological Critique," *Preventive Medicine* 42, no. 1 (January 2006): 4–13.

9. Z. Krivosikova et al., "The Association Between High Plasma Homocysteine Levels and Lower Bone Mineral Density in Slovak Women: The Impact of Vegetarian Diet," *European Journal of Nutrition* 49, no. 3 (October 7, 2009): 3147–53; C. Antoniades et al., Homocysteine and Coronary Atherosclerosis: From Folate Fortification to the Recent Clinical Trials," *European Heart Journal* 30, no. 1 (Jan 2009): 6–15.

10. J. E. Kerstetter et al., "Low Protein Intake: The Impact on Calcium and Bone Homeostasis in Humans," *Journal of Nutrition* 133, no. 3 (March 2003): 855S–61S.

11. A. Mithal et al., "Impact of Nutrition on Muscle Mass, Strength, and Performance in Older Adults," *Osteoporosis International* 24, no. 5 (December 18, 2012): 1555–66.

12. D. J. Millward "Sufficient Protein for Our Elders?," *American Journal of Clinical Nutrition* 88, no. 5 (November 2008): 1187–88; E. Gaffney-Stomberg et al., "Increasing Dietary Protein Requirements in Elderly People for Optimal Muscle and Bone Health," *Journal of the American Geriatric Society* 57, no. 6 (June 2009): 1073–79; W. W. Campbell et al., "The Recommended Dietary Allowance for Protein May Not Be Adequate for Older People to Maintain Skeletal Muscle," *Journal of Gerontology A Biological Science Medical Sciences* 56, no. 6 (June 2001): M373–80; D. K. Houston et al., "Dietary Protein Intake Is Associated with Lean Mass Change in Older, Community-Dwelling Adults: The Health, Aging, and Body Composition (Health ABC) Study, *American Journal of Clinical Nutrition* 87, no. 1 (January 2008): 150–55; D. Scott et al., "Associations Between Dietary Nutrient Intake and Muscle Mass and Strength in Community-Dwelling Older Adults: The Tasmanian Older Adult Cohort Study," *Journal of the American Geriatric Society* I58, no. 11 (Nov 2010): 2129–34.

13. Houston et al., "Dietary Protein."

14. R. G. Munger et al., "Prospective Study of Dietary Protein Intake and Risk of Hip Fracture in Postmenopausal Women," *American Journal of Clinical Nutrition* 69, no. 1 (1999): 147–52; J. H. Promislow et al., "Protein Consumption and Bone Mineral Density in the Elderly: The Rancho Bernardo Study," *American Journal of Epidemiology* 155, no. 7 (April 1 2002): 63–44; A. Devine et al., "Protein Consumption Is an Important Predictor off Lower Limb Bone Mass in Elderly Women," *American Journal of Clinical Nutrition* 81, no. 6 (June 2005): 1423–28.

15. D. L. Thorpe et al., "Effects of Meat Consumption and Vegetarian Diet on Risk of Wrist Fracture over 25 Years in a Cohort of Peri- and Postmenopausal Women," *Public Health Nutrition* 6 (August 9, 2007): 564–72.

16. Munger et al., "Prospective Study."

17. E. L. Knight et al., "The Impact of Protein Intake on Renal Function Decline in Women with Normal Renal Function or Mild Renal Insufficiency," *Annals of Internal Medicine* 18, no. 6 (March 18, 2003): 460–67.

18. H. A. Oboh et al., "Effect of Soaking, Cooking and Germination on the Oligosaccharide Content of Selected Nigerian Legume Seeds," *Plant Foods for Human Nutrition* 55, no. 2 (2000): 97–110.

19. V. C. Aries et al., "The Effect of a Strict Vegetarian Diet on the Faecal Flora and Faecal Steroid Concentration." *Journal of Pathology* 103 (1971): 54–56.

20. B. M. Tang et al., "Use of Calcium or Calcium in Combination with Vitamin D Supplementation to Prevent Fractures and Bone Loss in People Aged 50 Years and Older: A Meta-Analysis," *The Lancet* 370, no. 9588 (August 25, 2007): 657–66; H. A. Bischoff-Ferrari et al., "Effect of Calcium Supplementation on Fracture Risk: A Double-Blind Randomized Controlled Trial," *American Journal of Clinical Nutrition* 87, no. 6 (June 2008): 1945–51; R. L. Prince et al., "Effects of Calcium Supplementation on Clinical Fracture and Bone Structure: Results of a 5-Year, Double-Blind, Placebo-Controlled Trial in Elderly Women," *Archives of Internal Medicine* 166, no. 8 (April 24, 2006):869–75.

21. H. A. Bischoff-Ferrari et al., "Effect of Vitamin D on Falls: A Meta-Analysis." *JAMA* 291, no. 16 (April 28, 2004): 1999–2006.

22. T. J. Wang et al., "Vitamin D Deficiency and Risk of Cardiovascular Disease," *Circulation* 117, no. 4 (January 29, 2008): 503–11.

23. A. G. Pittas et al., "The Role of Vitamin D and Calcium in Type 2 Diabetes: A Systematic Review and Meta-Analysis," *Journal of Clinical Endocrinol Metabolism* 92, no. 6 (June 2007): 2017–29.

24. D. M. Freedman et al., "Prospective Study of Serum Vitamin D and Cancer Mortality in the United States," *Journal of the National Cancer Institute* 99, no. 21 (November 7, 2007): 1594–1602.

25. K. L. Munger et al., "Serum 25-hydroxyvitamin D Levels and Risk of Multiple Sclerosis," *JAMA* 296, no. 23 (December 20, 2006): 2832–38.

26. C. Oudshoorn et al., "Higher Serum Vitamin D_3 Levels Are Associated with Better Cognitive Test Performance in Patients with Alzheimer's Disease," *Dementia and Geriatr Cognitive Disorders* 25, no. 6 (20086):539–43.

27. Y. Milaneschi et al., "The Association Between Low Vitamin D and Depressive Disorders," *Molecular Psychiatry* (Apr 9, 2013).

28. A. C. Looker et al., "Prevalence of Low Femoral Bone Density in Older U.S. Adults from NHANES III," *Journal of Bone and Mineral Research* 12, no. 11 (November 1997): 1761–68.

29. M. F. Holick et al., "Age, Vitamin D, and Solar Ultraviolet," *The Lancet*, 2, no. 8671 (November 4, 1989;): 1104–5; A. G. Need et al., "Effects of Skin Thickness, Age, Body Fat, and Sunlight on Serum 25-hydroxyvitamin D," *American Journal of Clinical Nutrition* 58, no. 6 (December 1993): 882–85.

30. T. L. et al., "Increased Skin Pigment Reduces the Capacity of Skin to Synthesise Vitamin D_3," *The Lancet* 1, no. 8263 (January 9, 1982): 74–76.

31. C. A. Nowson and C. Margerison, "Vitamin D Intake and Vitamin D Status of Australians," *Medical Journal of Australia* 177, no. 3 (August 5, 2002): 149–52; N. Binkley et al., "Low Vitamin D Status Despite Abundant Sun Exposure," *Journal of Clinical Endocrinol Metabolism* 92, no. 6 (June 2007): 2130–35; E. T. Jacobs et al., "Vitamin D Insufficiency in Southern Arizona," *American Journal of Clinical Nutrition* 87, no. 3 (March 2008): 608–13.

32. M. F. Holick et al., "Vitamin D_2 Is as Effective as Vitamin D_3 in Maintaining Circulating Concentrations of 25-hydroxyvitamin D," *Journal of Clinical Endocrinol Metabolism* 93, no. 3

(March): 677–81, P. B. et l., "Effect of Vitamins D_2 and D_3 Supplement Use on Serum 25OHD Concentration in Elderly Women in Summer and Winter," *Calcified Tissue International* 74, no. 2 (February 2004;): 150–56.

33. J. W. Anderson et al., "Health Benefits of Dietary Fiber, *Nutrition Review* 67, no. 4 (April 2009): 188–205.

34. A. Santacruz et al., "Interplay Between Weight Loss and Gut Microbiota Composition in Overweight Adolescents," *Obesity (Silver Spring)* 16, no. 10 (October 2009): 1906–15.

35. P. Fischer-Posovszky et al., "Resveratrol Regulates Human Adipocyte Number and Function in a Sirt1–Dependent Manner," *American Journal of Clinical Nutrition* 82, no. 1 (July 2010): 5–15.

36. L. J. Appel et al., "A Clinical Trial of the Effects of Dietary Patterns on Blood Pressure: DASH Collaborative Research Group," *New England Journal of Medicine* 336, no. 16 (1997): 1117–24.

37. R. J. Barnard et al., "Diet and Exercise in the Treatment of NIDDM: The Need for early emphasis," *Diabetes Care* 17, no. 12 (December 1994): 1469–72.

38. K. M. Flegal et al., "Association of All-Cause Mortality with Overweight and Obesity Using Standard Body Mass Index Categories: A Systematic Review and Meta-Analysis," *JAMA* 309, no. 1 (January 2, 2013): 71–82.

39. M. Hamer and E. Stamatakis, "Metabolically Healthy Obesity and Risk of All-Cause and Cardiovascular Disease Mortality," *Journal of Clinical Endocrinol Metabolism* 97, no.7 (April 16, 2012): 2482–8.

40. L. Bacon et al., "Size Acceptance and Intuitive Eating Improve Health for Obese, Female Chronic Dieters," *Journal of the American Dietary Association* 105, no. 6 (June 2005;): 929–36.

CHAPTER 6. VEGAN DIETS FOR LIFELONG HEALTH

1. R. H.Knopp, X. Zhu, and B. Bonet, "Effects of Estrogens on Lipoprotein Metabolism and Cardiovascular Disease in Women," *Atherosclerosis* 110 (October 1994): S83–S91.

2. G. E. Fraser, "Vegetarian Diets: What Do We Know of Their Effects on Common Chronic Diseases? *American Journal of Clinical Nutrition* 89, no. 5 (May 2009): 1607S–12S.

3. L. Bissoli et al., "Effect of Vegetarian Diet on Homocysteine Levels," *Annals of Nutrition and Metabolism* 46, no. 2 (2002;): 73–79; S. G. De Biase et al., "Vegetarian Diet and Cholesterol and Triglycerides Levels, *Arquivos Brasileiros de Cardiologia* 88, no. 1 (January 2007): 35–39.

4. M. Krajcovicova-Kudlackova and P. Blazicek, "C-reactive Protein and Nutrition, *Bratisl Lek Listy* 106 (2005): 345–47; M. Krajcovicova-Kudlackova et al., "Effects of Diet and Age on Oxidative Damage Products in Healthy Subjects," *Physiological Research* 7, no. 4 (2008): 647–51.

5. D. J. Jenkins et al., "The effect of a Plant-Based Low-Carbohydrate ("Eco-Atkins") Diet on Body Weight and Blood Lipid Concentrations In Hyperlipidemic Subjects," *Archives of Internal Medicine* 169, no. 11 (June 8, 2009): 1046–54.

6. M. Valachovicova et al., "No Evidence of Insulin Resistance in Normal Weight Vegetarians: A Case Control Study," *European Journal of Nutriyion* 45, no. 1 (February 2006;): 52–54; C. J. Hung et al., "Taiwanese Vegetarians Have Higher Insulin Sensitivity Than Omnivores," *British Journal of Nutrition* 95, no. 1 (January 2006): 129–35; L. M. Goff et al., "Veganism and Its Relationship with Insulin Resistance and Intramyocellular Lipid. *European Journal of Clinical Nutrition* 59, no. 2 (February 2005): 291–98.

7. S. Tonstad et al., "Type of Vegetarian Diet, Body Weight, and Prevalence of Type 2 Diabetes," *Diabetes Care* 32, no. 5 (May 2009):791–96.

8. N. D. Barnard et al. A Low-Fat Vegan Diet and a Conventional Diabetes Diet in the Treatment of Type 2 Diabetes: A Randomized, Controlled, 74-Wk Clinical Trial," *American Journal of Clinical Nutrition* 89, no. 5 (May 2009): 1588S–96S.

9. H. Kahleova et al., "Vegetarian Diet Improves Insulin Resistance and Oxidative Stress Markers More Than Conventional Diet in Subjects with Type 2 Diabetes," *Diabetic Medicine* 28, no. 5 (May 2011): 549–59.

10. D. Ornish et al. "Changes in Prostate Gene Expression in Men Undergoing an Intensive Nutrition and Lifestyle Intervention," *Proceedings of the National Academy of Sciences (USA)* 105, no, 24 (June 17, 2008): 8369–74.

11. E. H. Haddad and J. S. Tanzman, "What Do Vegetarians in the United States Eat?," *American Journal of Clinical Nutrition* 78, no. 3 (September 2003): 626S–32S.

12. Y. Tantamango-Bartley et al., "Vegetarian Diets and the Incidence of Cancer in a Low-Risk Population," *Cancer Epidemiology, Biomarkers, & Prevention* 22, no. 2 (November 20, 2012): 286–94.

13. A. C. Sartori et al., "The Impact of Inflammation on Cognitive Function in Older Adults: Implications for Healthcare Practice and Research," *Journal of Neuroscience Nursing* 44, no. 4 (August 2012): 206–17; J. A. Luchsinger, S. Shea, and R. Mayeux, "Hyperinsulinemia and Risk of Alzheimer Disease," *Neurology* 63, no. 7 (October 12, 2004): 1187–92; E. Duron and O. Hanon, "Vascular Risk Factors, Cognitive Decline, and Dementia," *Vascular Health Risk Management* 4, no. 2 (2008): 363–81.

14. M. C. Morris et al., "Dietary Fats and the Risk of Incident Alzheimer Disease," *Archives of Neurolology* 60, no. 2 (February 2003): 194–200; S. A. Smith-Warner et al., "Types of Dietary Fat and Breast Cancer: A Pooled Analysis of Cohort Studies," *International Journal of Cancer* 92, no. 5 (June 1, 2001): 767–74; J. Wang et al., "Dietary Fat, Cooking Fat, and Breast Cancer Risk in a Multiethnic Population," *Nutrition and Cancer* 60, no. 4 (2008): 492–504; B. Vessby et al., "Substituting Dietary Saturated for Monounsaturated Fat Impairs Insulin Sensitivity in Healthy Men and Women: The KANWU Study," *Diabetologia* 44, no. 3 (March 2001): 312–9; F. B. Hu Ret al., "Diet and Risk of Type II Diabetes: The Role of Types of Fat and Carbohydrate," *Diabetologia* 44, no. 7 (July 2001): 805–17.

15. J. Hu et al., "Dietary Cholesterol Intake and Cancer," *Annals of Oncology* 23, no. 3 (February 2012): 491–500.

16. R. C. Shah et al., "Relation of Hemoglobin to Level of Cognitive Function in Older Persons," *Neuroepidemiology* 31, no. 1 (2009): 40–46; M. A. Lovell et al., "Copper, Iron and Zinc in Alzheimer's Disease Senile Plaques," *Journal of Neurological Science* 158, no. 1 (June 11, 1998): 47–52.

17. M. H. Kim and Y. J. Bae, "Postmenopausal Vegetarians' Low Serum Ferritin Level May Reduce the Risk for Metabolic Syndrome," *Biological Trace Element Research* 149, no. 1 (April 25, 2012): 34–41.

18. K. D. Burroughs et al., "Insulin-like Growth Factor-I: A Key Regulator of Human Cancer Risk?" [editorial] *Journal of the National Cancer Institute* 91, no. 7 (1999): 579–81.

19. N. E. Allen et al., "Hormones and Diet: Low Insulin-like Growth Factor-I but Normal Bioavailable Androgens in Vegan Men," *British Journal of Cancer* 83, no. 1 (2000): 95–97.

20. J. M. Chan et al., "Dairy Products, Calcium, and Prostate Cancer Risk in the Physicians' Health Study," *American Journal of Clinical Nutrition* 74, no. 4 (October 2001): 549–54.

21. R. A. Koeth et al., "Intestinal Microbiota Metabolism of l-carnitine, a Nutrient in Red Meat, Promotes Atherosclerosis," *National Medicine* 19, no. 5 (April 7, 2013): 576–85.

22. M. H. Carlsen et al., "The Total Antioxidant Content of More Than 3100 Foods, Beverages, Spices, Herbs and Supplements Used Worldwide," *Nutrition Journal* 9 (2010) : 3.

23. F. L. Crowe et al., "Fruit and Vegetable Intake and Mortality from Ischaemic Heart Disease: Results from the European Prospective Investigation into Cancer and Nutrition (EPIC)-Heart Study," *European Heart Journal* 32, no. 10 (May 2011): 1235–43.

24. M. Etminan, B. Takkouche, and F. Caamano-Isorna, "The Role of Tomato Products and Lycopene in the Prevention of Prostate Cancer: A Meta-Analysis of Observational Studies," *Cancer Epidemiology, Biomarkers, & Prevention* 13, no. 3 (March 2004): 340–45; H. S. Kim et al. "Effects of Tomato Sauce Consumption on Apoptotic Cell Death in Prostate Benign Hyperplasia and Carcinoma," *Nutrition and Cancer* 47, no. 1 (2003): 40–47.

25. J. Shi and M. Le Maguer, " Lycopene in Tomatoes: Chemical and Physical Properties Affected by Food Processing," *Critical Review of Biotechnology* 20, no. 4 (2000;): 293–334.

26. J. E. Cade JE, V. J. Burley, and D. C. Greenwood, "Dietary Fibre and Risk of Breast Cancer in the UK Women's Cohort Study," *International Journal of Epidemiology* 36, no. 2 (April 2007): 431–38; J. Y. Dong et al., "Dietary Fiber Intake and Risk of Breast Cancer: A Meta-Analysis of Prospective Cohort Studies," *American Journal of Clinical Nutrition* 94, no. 3 (July 20, 2011);900–5. M. C. Pike et al., "Estrogens, Progestogens, Normal Breast Cell Proliferation, and Breast Cancer Risk," *Epidemiology Review* 15, no. 1 (1993): 17–35.

27. V. G. Aries et al., "The Effect of a Strict Vegetarian Diet on the Faecal Flora and Faecal Steroid Concentration. *Journal of Pathology,* 103 (1972): 54–56.

28. M. M. Murphy, J. S. Douglass, and A. Birkett, "Resistant Starch Intakes in the United States," *Journal of the American Dietetic Association* 108, no. 1 (January 2008):67–78.

29. Y. Henrotin Y, B. Kurz B, and T. Aigner, "Oxygen and Reactive Oxygen Species in Cartilage Degradation: Friends or Foes?," *Osteoarthritis Cartilage* 13, no. 8 (August 2005): 643–54.

30. F. Blotman et al., "Efficacy and Safety of Avocado/Soybean Unsaponifiables in the Treatment of Symptomatic Osteoarthritis of the Knee and Hip: A Prospective, Multicenter, Three-Month, Randomized, Double-Blind, Placebo-Controlled Trial," *Revue du Rhumatisme English Edition* 64, 12 (Dec 1997): 825–34; T. E. Towheed et al, "Glucosamine Therapy for Treating Osteoarthritis," *Cochrane Database Syst Rev.* 2005(2):CD002946.

31. E. E. Kasim-Karakas et al., "Changes in Plasma Lipoproteins During Low-Fat, High-Carbohydrate Diets: Effects of Energy Intake," *American Journal of Clinical Nutrition* 71, no. 6 (2000): 1439–47; B. Lamarche, I. Lemieux, and J. P. Despres, "The Small, Dense LDL Phenotype and the Risk of Coronary Heart Disease: Epidemiology, Patho-Physiology and Therapeutic Aspects," *Diabetes & Metabolism* 25, no. 3 (1999): 199–211; S. Koba et al., "Significance of Small Dense Low-Density Lipoproteins and Other Risk Factors in Patients with Various Types of Coronary Heart Disease," *American Heart Journal* 144, no. 6 (December 2002): 1026–35.

32. D. J. Jenkins et al., "Nuts as a Replacement for Carbohydrates in the Diabetic Diet," *Diabetes Care,* 34, no. 8 (August 2011): 1706–11.

33. E. L. Richman EL, , et al., "Fat Intake After Diagnosis and Risk of Lethal Prostate Cancer and All-Cause Mortality," *JAMA Intern Medicine* (June 10 2013): 1–8.

34. J. Sabate, J. K. Oda, and E. Ros, "Nut Consumption and blood Lipid Levels: A Pooled Analysis of 25 Intervention Trials," *Archives of Internal Medicine* 170, no. 9 (May 10, 2010): 821–27.

35. J. H. Kelly Jr. and J. Sabate, "Nuts and Coronary Heart Disease: An Epidemiological Perspective," British Journal of Nutrition 96 (November 2006): S61–67.

36. E. Ros, "Nuts and Novel Biomarkers of Cardiovascular Disease," American Journal of Clinical Nutrition 89, no. 5 (May 2009): 1649S–56S.

37. S. Salvini et al., "Daily Consumption of a High-Phenol Extra Virgin Olive Oil Reduces Oxidative DNA Damage in Postmenopausal Women," British Journal of Nutrition 95, no. 4 (April, 2006): 742–51; C. Razquin et al., "A 3 Years Follow-up of a Mediterranean Diet Rich in Virgin Olive Oil Is Associated with High Plasma Antioxidant Capacity and Reduced Body Weight Gain," European Journal Clin Nutrition 63, no. 1 (December, 2009;): 1387–93; M. Fito et al., "Anti-inflammatory Effect of Virgin Olive Oil in Stable Coronary Disease Patients: A Randomized, Crossover, Controlled Trial," European Journal of Clinical Nutrition 62, no. 4 (April 2008): 570–74; M. I. Covas, V. Konstantinidou, and M. Fito, "Olive oil and Cardiovascular Health," Journal of Cardiovascular Pharmacolology 54, no. 6 (December, 2009): 477–82.

38. C. E. O'Neil et al., " Nut Consumption Is Associated with Decreased Health Risk Factors for Cardiovascular Disease and Metabolic Syndrome in U.S. Adults: NHANES 1999–2004," Journal of the American College of Nutrition 30, no. 6 (December, 2011): 502–10; K. McManus L. Antinoro, and F. Sacks, "A Randomized Controlled Trial of a Moderate-Fat, Low-Energy Diet Compared with a Low Fat, Low-Energy Diet for Weight Loss in Overweight Adults," International Journal of Obesity Related Metabolic Disorders 25, no. 10 (October 2001): 1503–11.

39. E. Lopez-Garcia et al., "Consumption of Trans Fatty Acids Is Related to Plasma Biomarkers of Inflammation and Endothelial Dysfunction," Journal of Nutrition 135, no. 3 (March 2005): 562–66.

40. A. Accorsi-Neto et al., "Effects of Isoflavones on the Skin of Postmenopausal Women: A Pilot Study," Clinics (São Paulo) 64, no 6 (2009): 505–10; T. Izumi T, et al., "Oral Intake of Soy Isoflavone Aglycone Improves the Aged Skin of Adult Women, Journal of Nutritional Science and Vitaminology (Tokyo) 53, no. 1 (February 2007): 57–62.

41. M. Messina et al., "Early Intake Appears to Be the Key to the Proposed Protective Effects of Soy Intake Against Breast Cancer. Nutr Cancer 2009;61:792–8.

42. X. O. Shu et al., "Soy Food Intake and Breast Cancer Survival," JAMA 302, 22 (December 9, 2009): 2437–43; X. Kang et al., "Effect of Soy Isoflavones on Breast Cancer Recurrence and Death for Patients Receiving Adjuvant Endocrine Therapy. CMAJ 182, no. 17 (November 23, 2010): 1857–62; B. J. Caan et al., "Soy Food Consumption and Breast Cancer Prognosis," Cancer Epidemiology & Biomarkers Prevention 20, no. 5 (May 2011): 854–58; N. Guha et al., "Soy isoflavones and Risk of Cancer Recurrence in a Cohort of Breast Cancer Survivors: The Life After Cancer Epidemiology Study," Breast Cancer Research and Treatment 118, no.2 (November 2009): 395–405; S. J. Nechuta et al., "Soy Food Intake After Diagnosis of Breast Cancer and Survival: An In-Depth Analysis of Combined Evidence from Cohort Studies of US and Chinese Women," American Journal of Clinical Nutrition 96, no. 1 9 (July 2012): 123–32.

43. Nechuta et al., "Soy Food Intake."

44. L. Yan and E. L. Spitznagel, "Soy Consumption and Prostate Cancer Risk in Men: A Revisit of a Meta-Analysis. American Journal of clinical Nutrition 89, no. 4 (April 2009): 1155–63.

45. M. Hussain et al., "Soy Isoflavones in the Treatment of Prostate Cancer, Nutrition and Cancer 47, no. 2 (2003): 111–17; M. Joshi et al., "Effects of Commercially Available Soy Products

on PSA in Androgen-Deprivation-Naive and Castration-Resistant Prostate Cancer. *Southern Medical Journal* 104, no. 11 (November 2011;): 736–40.

46. S. H. Li et al., "Effect of Oral Isoflavone Supplementation on Vascular Endothelial Function in Postmenopausal Women: A Meta-Analysis of Randomized Placebo-Controlled Trials," *American Journal of Clinical Nutrrition* 91, no. 2 (February 2010): 480–86.

47. X. Zhang , et al., "Soy Food Consumption Is Associated with Lower Risk of Coronary Heart Disease in Chinese Women. *Journal of Nutr* 133, no. 9 (September 2003): 2874–78; S. Sasazuki, "Case-Control Study of Nonfatal Myocardial Infarction in Relation to Selected Foods in Japanese Men and Women," *Japanese Circulation Journal* 65, no. 3 (March 2001): 200–206.

48. P. C. Calder et al. Dietary Factors and Low-Grade Inflammation in Relation to Overweight and Obesity," *British Journal of Nutrition* 106 suppl. 3 (December 2011): S5–78.

49. L. L. Koppes J. M. et al., "Moderate alcohol Consumption Lowers the Risk of Type 2 Diabetes: A Meta-Analysis of Prospective Observational Studies," *Diabetes Care* 28, no. 3 (March 2005): 719–725.

50. E. Linos E, M. D. Holmes, and W. C. Willett WC., "Diet and Breast Cancer," *Current Oncology Reports* 9, no. 1 (January 2007): 31–41.

51. T.A. Pearson et al. Markers of inflammation and Cardiovascular Disease: Application to Clinical and Public Health Practice: A Statement for Healthcare Professionals from the Centers for Disease Control and Prevention and the American Heart Association. *Circulation* 107, no. 3 (January 28, 2003): 499–511; M. J. Franz et al., "Evidence-Based Nutrition Principles and Recommendations for the Treatment and Prevention of Diabetes and Related Complications," *Diabetes Care* 25, no. 1 (January 2002): 148–98.

52. J. E. Manson et al., "A Prospective Study of Walking as Compared with Vigorous Exercise in the Prevention of Coronary Heart Disease in Women," *New England Journal of Medicine* 341, no. 9 (August 26, 1999): 650–58.

53. K. Yamamoto K et al., "Poor Trunk Flexibility Is Associated with Arterial Stiffening," *American Journal of Physiology Heart Circulation Physiology* 297, no. 4 (October 2009): H1314–18.

54. W. W. Campbell "Synergistic Use of Higher-Protein Diets or Nutritional Supplements with Resistance Training to Counter Sarcopenia," *Nutrition Revieew* 65, no. 9 (September 2007): 416–22.

55. R. K. et al. "Neurobiology of Exercise," *Obesity (Silver Spring)* 13, no. 3 (March 2006): 345–56.

56. S. J. Colcombe et al., "Aerobic Exercise Training Increases Brain Volume in Aging Humans," *Journal of Gerontology A Bioliological Science Medical Sciience* 61, no. 11 (November 2006): 1166–70.

57. S. Rovio et al., "Leisure-time Physical Activity at Midlife and the Risk of Dementia and Alzheimer's Disease, " *The Lancet Neurology* 4, no. 11 (November 2005:705–11; E. B. Larson et al., "Exercise Is Associated with Reduced Risk for Incident Dementia Among Persons 65 Years of Age and Older," *Annals of Internal Medicine* 144, no. 2 (January 17, 2006): 73–81.

58. S. K. Lutgendorf et al.," Life Stress, Mood Disturbance, and Elevated Interleukin-6 in Healthy Older Women," *Journal of Gerontolology A Biological Science Medical Science* 54, no. 9 (September 1999): M434–39.

59. B. S. McEwen, "Stress and Hippocampal Plasticity," *Annual Review of Neusscience* 22 (1999): 105–22.

60. M. L. Kohut et al., "Aerobic Exercise, but Not Flexibility/Resistance Exercise, Reduces Serum IL-18, CRP, and IL-6 Independent of Beta-Blockers, BMI, and Psychosocial Factors in Older Adults," *Brain, Behavior, and Immunity* 20, no. 3 (May 2006): 201–9.

61. J. A. Pasco et al., "Association of High-Sensitivity C-Reactive Protein with de Novo Major Depression," *British Journal of Psychiatry* 197, no. 5 (November 2010): 372–7.

62. R. J. Davidson et al., "Alterations in Brain and Immune Function Produced by Mindfulness Meditation," *Psychosomatic Medicine* 65, no. 4 (July–August 2003): 564–70.

63. *V. A. Barnes and D. W. Orme-Johnson, "Prevention and Treatment of Cardiovascular Disease in Adolescents and Adults Through the Transcendental Meditation Program: A Research Review Update," Current Hypertension Reviews 8, no. 3 (August 2012): 227–42.*

64. T. W. Pace et al., "Effect of Compassion Meditation on Neuroendocrine, Innate Immune and Behavioral Responses to Psychosocial Stress," *Psychoneuroendocrinology* 34, no. 1 (January 2009): 87–98.

INDEX

Page numbers in *italics* refer to tables.

ABOUT THE AUTHORS

Carol J. Adams is the author of the pioneering *The Sexual Politics of Meat*, called a "vegan bible" by *The New York Times* and now in a twentieth-anniversary edition, plus more than twenty other books and over one hundred articles. She frequently speaks on college campuses. She is working on a memoir about her decade as a caregiver. She lives near Dallas, Texas, with her partner and their two rescued dog companions, Holly and Inky. Find out more about Carol at caroljadams.com.

Patti Breitman is the director of the Marin Vegetarian Education Group and a cofounder of Dharma Voices for Animals. She is the coauthor, with Connie Hatch, of *How to Say No Without Feeling Guilty* and, with Carol J. Adams, of *How to Eat Like a Vegetarian Even If You Never Want to Be One*. Patti is on the advisory council of the Animals and Society Institute and grows vegetables in her community garden. She teaches seasonal vegan cooking classes in Marin County, California, where she lives.

Virginia Messina, MPH, RD, is coauthor of *Vegan for Life* and *Vegan for Her* and of the first textbook on vegetarian nutrition for medical professionals. She writes and speaks on vegan nutrition for both consumers and health professionals. Ginny serves on the advisory board of the Vegetarian Resource Group and on the board of directors of VegFund. She lives in Port Townsend, Washington, with her husband and an ever-changing population of rescued cats. Find out more about Ginny at TheVeganRD.com.

NeverTooLatetoGoVegan.com